Promoting Young People's Sexual Health

Across the world, heated debates arise as to the most suitable means of addressing the sexual health of young people. On one side are those who believe that keeping quiet about the issues will prevent experimentation and early sexual activity. On the other side are those who argue that young people have entitlements to information and services and that these are associated with safer outcomes.

Promoting Young People's Sexual Health reveals the complexity of the issues involved in this debate and demonstrates that there are no simple answers. Drawing on a wide range of literature and covering a wide range of areas, the book discusses:

- how young people's sexual activities are affected by the wider contexts in which they live;
- the practical and ideological barriers that constrain and inhibit the improvement of young people's sexual health at educational and service levels;
- some examples of innovative efforts to overcome some of these barriers;
- possible ways forward in terms of policy and legislative changes;
- how those in positions of authority to make policy and programmatic decisions need to accept their responsibilities more fully.

This book will appeal to students of sociology, anthropology, psychology, community and public health, as well as health and social care professionals. It is also essential reading for workers in the field of sexual health and HIV.

Roger Ingham is Director of the Centre for Sexual Health Research at the University of Southampton, UK, and an advisor to the UK Government's Teenage Pregnancy Unit.

Peter Aggleton is Director of the Thomas Coram Research Unit at the Institute of Education, University of London, UK.

Sexuality, Culture and Health series

Edited by Peter Aggleton, Institute of Education, University of London, UK
Richard Parker, Columbia University, New York, USA
Sonia Correa, ABIA, Rio de Janeiro, Brazil
Gary Dowsett, La Trobe University, Melbourne, Australia
Shirley Lindenbaum, City University of New York, USA

This new series of books offers cutting-edge analysis, current theoretical perspectives and up-to-the-minute ideas concerning the interface between sexuality, public health, human rights, culture and social development. It adopts a global and interdisciplinary perspective in which the needs of poorer countries are given equal status to those of richer nations. The books are written with a broad range of readers in mind, and will be invaluable to students, academics and those working in policy and practice. The series also aims to serve as a spur to practical action in an increasingly globalised world.

Also available in the series:

Dying to be Men
Youth, masculinity and social exclusion
Gary T. Barker

Sex, Drugs and Young People
International perspectives
Edited by Peter Aggleton, Andrew Ball and Purnima Mane

Promoting Young People's Sexual Health

International perspectives

Edited by Roger Ingham and Peter Aggleton

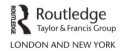

Routledge
Taylor & Francis Group

LONDON AND NEW YORK

First published 2006
by Routledge
2 Park Square, Milton Park, Abingdon, Oxon OX14 4RN

Simultaneously published in the USA and Canada
by Routledge
270 Madison Ave, New York, NY 10016

Routledge is an imprint of the Taylor & Francis Group, an informa business

Typeset in Sabon by
GreenGate Publishing Services, Tonbridge, Kent
Printed and bound in Great Britain by
T. J. International Ltd., Padstow, Cornwall

British Library Cataloguing in Publication Data
A catalogue record for this book is available from the British Library

Library of Congress Cataloging in Publication Data
Promoting young people's sexual health : international perspectives /
edited by Roger Ingham and Peter Aggleton.
      p. ; cm. — (Sexuality, culture and health)
   Includes bibliographical references and index.
      ISBN 0–415–37482–0 (hardback) — ISBN 0–415–37483–9 (pbk.)
1. Health behavior in adolescence. 2. Youth—Sexual behavior.
3. Hygiene, Sexual. I. Ingham, Roger, 1945- II. Aggleton, Peter. III. Series:
Sexuality, culture and health series. [DNLM: 1. Sexual Behavior—psychology. 2. Adolescent Behavior. 3. Adolescent. 4. Health Policy. 5. Sex
Education. WS 462 P9655 2006]
   RJ47.53.P76 2006
   613'.0433—dc22
                                                        2006010347

ISBN10: 0–415–37482–0 (hbk)
ISBN10: 0–415–37483–9 (pbk)

ISBN13: 978–0–415–37482–8 (hbk)
ISBN13: 978–0–415–37483–5 (pbk)

Contents

Illustrations

Tables

Figures

Contributors

Peter Aggleton is Director of the Thomas Coram Research Unit at the Institute of Education, University of London. The author and editor of over twenty books in the field of health promotion, he has acted as a senior advisor and consultant to UNAIDS, UNESCO, UNICEF, WHO and a wide range of other international agencies.

Mohamed M. Ali is a statistician in the Department of Reproductive Health and Research at WHO, conducting clinical trials and household surveys in reproductive health. Before joining WHO, he worked for several years at the Centre for Population Studies at the London School of Hygiene and Tropical Medicine. His current research interests include contraceptive use dynamics, mortality estimates and the application of multi-level modelling in health research.

Gary Barker is Executive Director of Instituto Promundo, a non-governmental organisation based in Rio de Janeiro, Brazil, that works to promote gender equality and health among young people and equitable community development. His doctorate is in child and adolescent development, and he has coordinated research and program development in gender socialisation and sexual and reproductive health in Latin America, the Caribbean, Africa, Asia and North America.

Paul Boyce is an ESRC post-doctoral research fellow at the Thomas Coram Research Unit, Institute of Education, University of London. His research interests include male-to-male sexuality in India, gender theory, anthropology and international HIV/AIDS policy.

Joanna Busza is a lecturer in sexual and reproductive health at the London School of Hygiene and Tropical Medicine. Her research focuses on the design and evaluation of community-based health interventions. Joanna also works with non-governmental organisations in developing countries to develop appropriate monitoring and evaluation strategies for sexual and reproductive health projects with vulnerable populations.

Elaine Chase is a research officer at the Thomas Coram Research Unit, Institute of Education, University of London. Her work, both in the UK and internationally, focuses on the health and wellbeing of children and young people, in particular those who are marginalised and disadvantaged.

John Cleland is Professor of Medical Demography at the London School of Hygiene and Tropical Medicine. His special interests include the study of sexual behaviour, contraceptive use and condom use in Asia and Africa.

Martine Collumbien is a lecturer in sexual health research at the London School of Hygiene and Tropical Medicine. Her work focuses on social and cultural aspects of sexual health and the use of research evidence in social marketing programmes.

Megan Douthwaite was a research fellow at the London School of Hygiene and Tropical Medicine and currently works as freelance consultant. She has extensive research experience in the monitoring and evaluation of sexual and reproductive health programmes for young people in South and Southeast Asia.

Roger Ingham is Professor of Health and Community Psychology at the University of Southampton, where he also directs the Centre for Sexual Health Research. He has extensive experience of research and national and international policy involvement in the area of young people's sexual health.

Laboni Jana is Assistant Director at the Child In Need Institute (CINI), a nationally recognised NGO in India. A public health professional by training, Laboni has been working in the area of reproductive and sexual health for the last ten years, with a focus on building evidence-based programme approaches with young people.

Eleanor King is a research assistant at Imperial College, London. She worked in Australia on the National Needle and Syringe Programme where she also completed an immunological laboratory project as part of an MSc in HIV/STIs.

Wendy Macdowall is a lecturer and MRC training fellow at the London School of Hygiene and Tropical Medicine. Her research interests include sex education, mass media and sexual health promotion and seasonal variations in sexual behaviour. She co-edited *Health Promotion Theory* (2005) and *Health Promotion Practice* (2006) both published by the Open University Press.

Cicely Marston is a lecturer in social science at the London School of Hygiene and Tropical Medicine. She is an interdisciplinary researcher. Her work has focused on behaviour theory, and on sexual and reproductive health, particularly of young people.

Susannah Mayhew is a lecturer in health policy and reproductive health at the London School of Hygiene and Tropical Medicine. Her research interests include health policy and systems issues relating to reproductive and sexual health in Africa and Asia.

Kirstin Mitchell is an ESRC/MRC doctoral candidate at the London School of Hygiene and Tropical Medicine. She has worked on HIV/AIDS and sexual health issues in Uganda and the UK since 1995. Her research interests include young people and communication, research methodology, and sexual dysfunction.

Julie Pulerwitz is Research Director of the Horizons Program at the Population Council/PATH, a global HIV/AIDS operations research program. Dr. Pulerwitz has worked in Asia, Latin America, and Africa, with a focus on behaviour change, gender and male involvement, HIV-related stigma, and indicator development.

Christine Ricardo is a senior program officer at Instituto Promundo and coordinates Program M, an international collaboration for the promotion of young women's empowerment and sexual and reproductive health. She has extensive experience working with organisations providing mentoring and other support services for women and children.

Valéria Rocha is a senior project officer at World Education, Inc. She has seven years of research experience in projects about women's health education, young people's behaviour and the family, gender and socio-economic development in the USA, Latin American and Asian countries.

Nicole Stone is a research fellow at the Centre for Sexual Health Research at the University of Southampton. She has worked in the field of young people's sexual health in both the UK and internationally since 1995. Her research interests include early sexual conduct, contraceptive use dynamics and service utilisation.

Ian Warwick is a senior research officer at the Thomas Coram Research Unit at the Institute of Education, University of London. He has carried out research in the fields of sexuality, HIV/AIDS, young people, health and education since 1986.

Kate Wood is a research associate of the Thomas Coram Research Unit, Institute of Education, University of London, and is currently studying medicine at the University of Bristol. Trained as a medical anthropologist, her doctorate involved ethnographic research on young people's lives and sexual health in a South African township, with a focus on sexual violence and responses to AIDS.

Acknowledgements

We would like to thank the UK Department of International Development for providing the funding for the *Safe Passages to Adulthood* programme. We would, in this connection, like to thank all those many individuals and agencies across the world who contributed in one way or another to the success of the programme. We hope that this volume will offer support to them in their often difficult and challenging work to improve the sexual health of young people.

We would also like to thank Sean Jennings and Fiona Thirlwell for their tremendous assistance with the editing of this book and other forms of support.

Roger Ingham, Southampton
Peter Aggleton, London

Introduction

Roger Ingham and Peter Aggleton

Some years ago, there was a major debate in the United Kingdom's House of Lords about whether sex education should be made a compulsory part of the school curriculum. Many and varied points of view were expressed – some for, some against, some in between – and various different angles were explored – for example, whether parents should have the right to withdraw their children from lessons on religious and/or cultural grounds, whether any coverage should be included as a separate topic, as part of biology or as part of personal and social education, what issues should be covered, and so on. This is not the place to describe the arguments or the outcomes. But two features of the debate were particularly notable.

First, the contributions of nearly all of the speakers could be readily categorised into one of two discourses, or sets of taken-for-granted assumptions. The first of these was the view that teaching, or telling, young people about sex and sexual matters would encourage them to go out and 'experiment' in inappropriate ways.

> It is no use preaching that the family is the natural unit of society and then doing something to undermine it. The needle, not normal sex, is the major source of AIDS
>
> (The Earl of Halsbury)

> … information on the kind of sex education that is being given in schools today is not just information; it encourages them to act on it. It affects their moral outlook, their moral behaviour and their conduct in general … it is not just information, it is an encouragement to promiscuity
>
> (Baroness Ellis)

> I believe that the real answer for dealing with AIDS is for the Government to take their courage in both hands and *tell* citizens that, if they want to avoid these diseases, they should be chaste before marriage and faithful within it
>
> (Lord Ashbourne)

The second was the view that education and support were essential in order to enable young people to protect themselves from regrettable outcomes, be they physical or psychological.

> In our society everything from coffee to cars is sold through sex appeal. Sexuality is part of our art and culture. We cannot avoid it ... therefore let us provide the facts ... I cannot think of any period in history when abstinence has been the norm ... I suggest that a more realistic approach is to provide information
>
> (Lord Addington)

> ... we have no right ... to deny children information which it may be essential for them to have to lead happy and healthy lives. Unless they have information and knowledge, they can fall into the trap of temptation which surrounds them. The temptations are far more powerful than the equipment that they have to resist them
>
> (Lord Houghton)

The second prominent feature of the debate was the way in which many of the speakers 'warranted' – or attempted to justify — their particular expertise to speak in the debate on one or more grounds. Some claimed their warrant through having been a teacher, some as having a medical background, some as being parents, some as being grandparents, some through the views of their own particular faiths, some as being young, some as having been young once, some as now being old and experienced, and so on.

Although this particular debate occurred in the somewhat rarefied atmosphere of the UK's upper chamber of government, similarly opposed arguments, as well as the efforts to justify particular expertise to talk about young people and sex, can be heard throughout every region of the world. In parliament, in school governors' meetings, in health policy decision-making fora, in local communities, and in many other venues, such issues are debated, often heatedly, and inevitably with severe implications for the sexual health of young people. Many people in positions of influence, be they politicians, health workers, teachers, parents, and others, believe that they are 'experts' in the field.

For many a year, religion, cultural opinions and rhetoric were the only ways in which the dilemmas raised by young people's emerging sexuality – and the implications – could be resolved; research into the area was minimal, and those showing too much interest in the topic were treated with some suspicion. The emergence of HIV, however, had a radical impact on this climate. It became imperative that efforts were made to gain a clear understanding not only of what sorts of sexual activities were being engaged in, but also the factors that affected the nature of such activities in terms of safety and protection from unintended outcomes.

The early approaches to this challenge were focussed primarily on those who had initially been identified as being at particular risk from infection – the so-called 'risk groups'. Similarly, efforts were made to identify individuals who exhibited more risky behaviour than did others, and to explore aspects of their psychological attributes (knowledge, attitudes, perceptions, and so on) so that they could be targeted with appropriate interventions in order to correct their apparent 'deficits'.

As time has passed, however, and more penetrative research and conceptual and theoretical analyses have been developed, so this early emphasis on individual 'targeting' has been supplemented by much greater attention to other issues. The chapters in this book have been written to provide coverage of these more *contextual* ways of understanding the complex realities of young people's sexual development, and the implications of these for programmatic responses to the challenges that the world faces.

In Part One, the first two chapters cover some important methodological issues; first, Mohamed Ali and John Cleland consider the value of large surveys for assessing young people's sexual activity, and highlight some of the key problems that are inherent in their use. They propose that societal and cultural factors introduce bias into the responses; since the strength and form of these various biases will differ between countries, they cast some doubt on the value of survey data being used for cross-national comparisons. However, since the biases are likely to be consistent across time within a particular country, they suggest that trend data can be used to explore change; this approach is illustrated with some important data from countries in sub-Saharan Africa and South and Central America.

Next, Cicely Marston, Ellie King and Roger Ingham provide a summary of the value of using qualitative approaches better to understand aspects of young people's sexual activity; they argue that these should be used to supplement survey data rather than to replace them. Taking one specific example – that of some of the issues that influence condom use – they show how interviews and focus groups reveal a number of the key social and relationship influences. Further, there appear to be some commonalities across countries and regions in these factors; the clear message is that simply making condoms more available and accessible, and improving knowledge, will not alone lead to increased usage.

Roger Ingham next considers the concept of 'context' in relation to young people's sexual activity, and demonstrates that the sheer complexity of the situation renders it unlikely that any simple approaches to change will be effective. Young people live in complex social and physical environments, and these need to be taken fully into account; this approach encourages the shift away from a notion of individual risk-takers towards one of vulnerabilities and vulnerable situations. The role of 'adults' in creating and sustaining these contexts, needs to be explored more fully.

A key thread that has emerged over the past years of research is the importance of gender and gender relations in understanding sexual activity and sexuality. Christine Ricardo, Gary Barker, Julie Pulerwitz and Valéria Rocha consider this area, stressing that the field has moved on a long way from simply regarding 'gender' as being about women to an understanding that men – and notions of masculinities – are equally deserving of research and programmatic attention. They provide some exciting examples of programmes to increase young people's understandings of gender in its various forms that provide some hope for the future.

In Part Two, we move on to some areas of interest involving more specific groups of young people in especially vulnerable situations. Elaine Chase and Peter Aggleton discuss issues relevant to the sexual health of children and young people living on the streets. While acknowledging the genuine adversity that such young people face and the need for structural intervention to promote and sustain children's rights, they highlight the creativity and resourcefulness that can be tapped in young person-focused programmes and responses.

Next, Peter Aggleton, Ian Warwick and Paul Boyce consider the wide variety of forms of sexual attraction and the specific problems faced by same-sex attracted young people through stigma and the narrow assumptions made by others about them. These are issues rarely addressed in the international sexual health literature, where the assumption is often made that young people are (or should be) either non-sexual or heterosexual. As this chapter shows, in every region of the world, sexual diversity is as much a characteristic of those who are young as those who are older, and if they are to speak to real lives and circumstances, programmes must respond accordingly.

In the following chapter, Kate Wood covers the relationships between sexual violence and sexual health, revealing something of the intimate connections between these phenomena and existing gender relations. She highlights too the multiple meanings that sex and sexual relations can carry and the differential opportunities for women and for men to express their sexual interests and needs.

Finally in this same section, Joanna Busza considers the various forms of transactional sex and their linkages to health issues. She differentiates between different forms of prostitution and sex work, describing too the various transactional and/or compensated sexual relationships into which young people enter, consensually or otherwise. Her work raises important questions for those who would seek unproblematically to link all forms of sex work and transactional sex to exploitation and abuse.

Each of these chapters is challenging to read, and provides a clear insight into the realities of sexual activity and its many forms of manifestation across the world. In many countries, the existence of same-sex attraction, or of sexual violence, is strenuously denied and ignored; only once these realities are acknowledged by those in positions to respond can there be hope that genuine change might be forthcoming. Similarly, to make an outright condemnation of, for example, 'prostitution', and to coerce others into publicly condemning the practice through funding conditions, is to grossly oversimplify the contexts in which different forms of transactional sex occur, and is likely to lead to greater sexual health problems in the future.

Part Three contains four chapters that consider some different ways of responding to the challenges faced. Martine Collumbien, Megan Douthwaite and Laboni Jana discuss ways of evaluating whether, and how, programmatic interventions have an effect; crucially, they show how involving young people themselves in the evaluation process – rather than basing them on the notion that 'adults know best' – can in itself have highly positive benefits.

Wendy Macdowall and Kirstin Mitchell discuss the role and potential of the mass media as agents of change in relation to social norms, and as providers of information in attractive and stimulating ways. Nicole Stone and Roger Ingham provide an overview of sex and relationships programming, and the need for this to be comprehensive in its coverage of information, skills and values. Finally, Roger Ingham and Susannah Mayhew cover some of the aspects involved in achieving change through influencing those in a position to change policy, whether this be policy at a high level (Policy with a big P) or at a more local family or community level (policy with a little p).

The impetus for this volume came from the *Safe Passages to Adulthood* programme, a major six-year programme of applied research supported by the UK Department for International Development. This was coordinated by Roger Ingham, Peter Aggleton and John Cleland, and brought together teams of multi-disciplinary researchers from the UK and across the world. Overall, more than 200 individuals and groups participated in the work in Africa, Asia, Australia, the Americas and Europe.[1]

All of the contributors to this volume are committed to the importance of good and reliable research to explore the complex nature of young people and their sexual health. Equally, they are all committed to a rights-based approach to work within this field. Since the majority of the emerging research supports the general direction of a rights-based approach, no conflict arises. The conflict, whether they realise it or not, and whether they accept it or not, lies with those who refuse to accept the reality of young people's sexual development and the challenges – some more immense than others – that they face. From this perspective, one needs to ask 'who are the real risk-takers?'.

Note

1   Further information on the programme and its outputs can be found at <www.socstats.soton.ac.uk/cshr/SafePassages>

Part I

Chapter 1

Uses and abuses of surveys on the sexual behaviour of young people

Mohamed M. Ali and John Cleland

Introduction

Until the late 1980s, the interest of many social scientists in sexual behaviour was restricted to the context of marriage. Malinowski (1929) and Mead (1949) are among the minority of anthropologists who regarded sexuality and social control of sexual expression as legitimate domains of study. Similarly, demographers have had a longstanding interest in sexual behaviour, but mainly as a determinant of fertility. Questions on post-natal abstinence have been a standard feature of demographic enquiries in Africa since the World Fertility Survey (WFS) in the 1970s. This information has proved crucial in attempts to understand reproductive regimes in that region (for example, Lestheaghe, 1989). Parenthetically, the custom of prolonged post-natal abstinence in West Africa has now emerged as a powerful influence on the extra-marital sexual activities of husbands with potentially serious consequences for disease transmission (Cleland *et al.*, 1999).

Frequency of coitus between marriage partners has also been studied by demographers. The interest here has been on the probability of conception, one of the proximate determinants of fertility about which we know least. In family planning research, also, coital frequency within marriage has proved relevant to the assessment of the effectiveness of different contraceptive methods (for example, Westoff, 1974).

The advent of the HIV pandemic has transformed research priorities. In most developing countries, the main route of infection is heterosexual intercourse and the strongest individual risk factor is the number of sexual partners. The majority of infections occur among young people. Thus the focus of attention had to shift away from sexual behaviour within marriage (though this aspect remains important) to sexual partnerships before or outside of marriage, in order to understand the spread of the disease, inform public information campaigns and evaluate interventions to check the spread of epidemics.

This chapter concerns the potential contribution that surveys – the collection of information from samples by standardised questionnaires or equivalent – can make to the study of the sexual behaviour of young people, in the era of HIV/AIDS. By young people, we have in mind primarily persons who are between puberty and marriage, although few surveys canvass individuals below the age of 15 years. In most countries of the world, the average age at first marriage (or first cohabiting partnership) has risen, thereby lengthening the phase in which people may be sexually active without full social approval.

Doubt is often expressed about the willingness of young people to divulge details of their sex lives to a stranger. An analogy with fertility and family planning surveys is appropriate. In the 1960s and early 1970s, study of the topic was dominated by Knowledge, Attitudes and Practice (KAP) surveys, that varied in quality, coverage and content. Their results were greeted with considerable scepticism. For instance, it was doubted that individuals would be prepared to reveal intimate details about their contraceptive habits. Partly in response, the WFS was created in 1972 to conduct mutually comparable high quality surveys in developing countries. The WFS restored the credibility of the survey method and much of our knowledge about fertility, childhood mortality and their determinants comes from this programme and its successor, the Demographic and Health Surveys (DHS) project. Over 50 developing countries have now conducted at least two high quality, representative surveys, thus permitting analysis of trends in vital rates in addition to cross-sectional differentials. Surveys have proved indispensable in monitoring progress towards policy goals concerning child survival and reproductive control.

It is now accepted that high quality large-scale surveys yield dependable evidence on contraception, and related aspects of behaviour. However, the record is not one of unalloyed success. The survey method, in most countries, has proved inadequate at overcoming resistance to the reporting of induced abortion, a procedure that is both illegal and stigmatised in many developing countries (Barreto *et al.,* 1992).

Has the willingness of respondents to report non-marital sexual partners proved more similar to the example of contraception or to that of abortion? This big question is addressed later in the chapter. Such concerns, however, did not for a moment deter the HIV/AIDS movement from enthusiastic promulgation of sexual behaviour surveys. Coordinated programmes of survey research were initiated by the then Global Programme on AIDS at the World Health Organisation for Asia, Latin America and Africa in the late 1980s (Cleland and Ferry, 1995) and many industrialised countries undertook similar surveys (Hubert *et al.,* 1998). Since then other survey programmes have started. The Centers for Disease Control in Atlanta, USA (www.cdc.gov) have sponsored youth surveys with an equal emphasis on reproduction and sexual behaviour; the geographical focus has been on Central Asia and Latin America. Family Health International (www.fhi.org) has funded many behavioural surveillance surveys, often concentrating on high-risk groups but also including India's very large 2001 national survey on youth (National AIDS Control Organisation, India and UNICEF, 2002). The Demographic and Health Survey (www.measuredhs.com) project for the last decade or so has incorporated questions on pre- and extra-marital partnerships in most of its surveys. Population Services International (www.psi.org), the leading condom social marketing organisation, has conducted innumerable surveys on risky sex and condom use.

While the contents of these centrally coordinated programmes vary, they are increasingly influenced by a set of internationally agreed behavioural indicators, by which progress towards achievement of the goals of HIV-prevention campaigns can be monitored. Monitoring of major international initiatives often focuses on a limited set of indicators. In the case of HIV, these include the Millennium Development Goals (which have one sexual behaviour indicator – condom use at last sex with a higher-risk partner) and the goals set at the 2001 United Nations General Assembly Special Session (UNGASS) on AIDS. The list of UNAIDS core behavioural indicators relevant to young people are listed in Table 1.1. The rationale for most of the

Table 1.1 UNAIDS Indicators for young people

Indicator	Denominator	Numerator
Median age at first sex	The age by which 50% of young people aged 15–24 say they have already had sex	All young people
Pre-marital sex in last year	All young people who have never had a cohabiting partner	Young people who have never had a cohabiting partner and who had sex in the last year
Condom use during pre-marital sex	All young sexually active people who have never had a cohabiting partner	Those who used a condom at their most recent sex
Multiple partners in last year	All young people	Young people who report more than one partner in last year
Condom use at last higher risk sex	All young people	Young people who used condom at the most recent sex with a non-cohabiting partner in the last year
Condom use at first sex	All young people who have ever had sex	Young people who used a condom the first time they had sex
Age mixing in sexual relationships	Women aged 15–19 who had sex with a man to whom they are not married in the last 12 months	Women aged 15–19 who had sex with a man to whom they are not married and who is 10 or more years older (based on their last three reported partnerships)

indicators lies in the distinction between presumptively lower-risk sexual partners (spouses or cohabiting partners) and higher-risk, non-cohabiting partners, and between condom use and non-use at most recent coital act with a higher-risk partner. Other rationales are that early sexual debut and sex with an older partner predispose towards high risk.

The relevance for disease transmission of these indicators varies by setting and epidemic phase. The match between indicators and HIV epidemiology is usually closest in the early and mid phases of generalised epidemics. In mature generalised epidemics, where an appreciable proportion of cohabiting couples are HIV discordant, transmission between cohabiting partners will make a large contribution to HIV incidence, thus undermining the equation of marital sex with low risk. Conversely in low-level and concentrated epidemics, the sexual conduct of the general population, or of youth, will be less relevant. Nevertheless, the UNAIDS core behavioural indicators correspond closely to the broad thrust of HIV prevention efforts aimed at the general population, and thus maintain their practical relevance regardless of epidemiological phase. Recent evidence shows that the behaviours represented by indicators are amenable to change. They are conceptually simple and relatively easy to measure. There is no reason to believe that their validity or reliability is lower than alternative measures. In view of the amount of expert input into their development, it is perhaps not surprising that they stand up well to critical scrutiny.

The centrally coordinated survey programmes have been accompanied by a plethora of more specialised, localised surveys, many of which have collected detailed information on sexual networks by obtaining a string of information on all sexual partners in the past 12 months. Imaginative adaptations of the classical face-to-face interview technique of developing country surveys have been devised. In Tanzania, for instance, the self-completion questionnaire approach has been modified for surveys of semi-literate teenage school students by reading out questions in a classroom context (Plummer et al., 2004). In Kenya, computer-assisted methods of data capture have been extended for use with young people of varying literacy by the computerised administration of questions though headphones rather than on the screen (Mensch et al., 2003; Hewett et al., 2004). In Zimbabwe, an ingenious confidential ballot box procedure has been used as an adjunct to conventional interviewing to elicit answers to particularly sensitive questions (Gregson et al., 2002, 2004). Diary methods have been adapted by repeated weekly interviews of a panel of informants, with day-by-day questions on sexual partners and sexual acts (Enel et al., 1994).

The common motivation behind most of these innovations is to increase anonymity and thereby lower the barriers to disclosure of socially disapproved behaviour. And, in general, the application of these techniques does result in higher estimates of multiple partnerships, and so on. But this apparent superiority over face-to-face interviews is not guaranteed. In Tanzania, self-administered questionnaires yielded similar results to interviews, though in-depth interviews suggested a much higher level of sexual networking (Plummer *et al.*, 2004). In exceptional cases, the innovations may be counterproductive. In Western Kenya, for example, audio-computer-assisted methods gave less plausible results than interviews, perhaps because the young persons were so unfamiliar with the technology and distrusted it (Mensch *et al.*, 2003). Moreover, these departures from normal survey procedures are not feasible for large surveys in poor countries. Self-completion questionnaires are well adapted to institutional study populations but inappropriate for community-based enquiries. Computer-assisted methods are prohibitively expensive for large investigations and the ballot box procedure poses logistical problems and requires highly trained interviewers. For this reason, no practical alternative exists to conventional face-to-face interviewing for most surveys of young people in poor countries.

Do face-to-face interviews with young people present problems that are not encountered in similar interviews of adults? Ethical considerations are certainly a key issue, particularly with regard to the age at which young persons can provide informed consent, thus obviating the need to seek parental consent. No internationally agreed rules exist on this vexed topic. Confidentiality is often of special importance, because disclosure of sexual activity could have serious repercussions. Reports of sexual coercion and abuse raise further ethical dilemmas and many surveys make provision for possible referral of extreme cases (Schenk and Williamson, 2005). In most other ways, surveys of the young differ little from those of older respondents.

Advances in the technology for collection of biological specimens has made possible another development – the integration of behavioural and biological measurement. The number of data sets that allow comparison of behavioural reports with laboratory evidence of infection with HIV or other sexually transmitted infections has increased substantially, most notably following the DHS decision to collect blood samples in most of its recent African surveys. At first, this combination of different types of data may appear to offer useful opportunities to validate self-reported behaviour. However, these opportunities are very limited in cross-sectional surveys. An individual with one lifetime partner may become infected with HIV, whereas someone with many partners may well remain uninfected. The complexities of the association between condom use and infection have led some unwary commentators to dismiss the protective efficacy of condoms. A positive association is often found but this will usually reflect one or both of two possibilities: either HIV was acquired before the initiation of condom use or condom users have more sexual partners than non-users and remain at higher risk because the device is not used with 100 percent consistency (Slaymaker and Zaba, 2003). Indeed one of the few clear-cut but still partial methods of validating behavioural reports by biological evidence is to assess the proportion of self-reported virgins who are infected (Cowan *et al.*, 2002).

A further major development, which initially came as a blow to survey practitioners, was the realisation that sexual behaviour, even if measured with apparent accuracy, can't explain why, in Africa, some countries experience explosive and devastatingly severe HIV epidemics while other countries remain relatively unscathed. The key study in this regard was the multi-disciplinary investigation of four cities – two with high HIV prevalence and two with stable low prevalence – sponsored by UNAIDS (Ferry *et al.*, 2001). Rather minor differences in sexual behaviour between cities were recorded and the implication is that biological factors (circumcision of men, co-infection with ulcerating sexual transmitted diseases or different HIV sub-types) probably account for much of the variation in epidemic spread.

How dependable are survey measures of sexual behaviour?

As noted above, opportunities to assess self-reported sexual behaviour against a gold-standard of truth are extremely limited. In industrialised countries where trends in abortions, teenage births and sexually transmitted infections are available, aggregate consistency with behavioural trends from repeated surveys can be assessed (for example, for U.S. teenagers, Biddlecom, 2004). In most developing countries, the possibilities for even this overall comparison are meagre; data on abortions and sexually transmitted infections are typically unavailable and reliable tracking of HIV is problematic even in countries with a surveillance system. Critiques of the quality of survey data on sexual behaviour must rely to an uncomfortable extent on criteria of coherence and plausibility, as well as drawing on the results of specialist methodological research.

Since the late 1980s, hundreds of surveys of sexual behaviour have been undertaken in developing countries. Over the same period, many methodological reviews and results of experimental research on different methods of investigation have been published (for example, Ankrah, 1989; Frank, 1994; Huygens *et al.*, 1996; Weinhardt *et al.*, 1998; Fenton *et al.*, 2001; Cleland *et al.*, 2004). The purpose of this section is to distil the main lessons from this mass of recent experience. Most of these lessons apply equally to surveys of youth and of adults.

The validity of survey responses concerning sexual behaviour depends primarily on three main conditions: understanding the questions, accuracy of recall, and willingness to report truthfully (Obeymeyer, 2005). All three are a common source of problems. The formal terms 'vaginal intercourse' or 'heterosexual partner' are prone to misunderstanding, even in Europe and USA (Binson and Catania, 1998). Recall of coital frequency over the past four weeks is inaccurate: response distributions often show heaping at multiples of four suggesting that respondents answer in terms of a week and then multiply (Blanc and Rutenberg, 1991). The same degree of inaccuracy no doubt applies to reported number of partners in the past 12 months for those respondents with more than a few such partners. But the greatest threat to validity stems from unwillingness to report truthfully and the rest of this section focuses on this key consideration.

The experience of the last 15 years suggests that willingness to disclose details of sexual conduct varies with social setting, sex of respondent, survey design and nature of information required.

Variation by *social setting* is to be expected because the social sanctions applied to sexual expression of young people are so diverse, from brutal enforcement of standards of chastity by honour killings in South Asia to widespread tolerance or even encouragement of sexual experimentation in other parts of the world. In general, of course, willingness to disclose 'illicit' sexual contact will be lowest in societies where it is (or thought to be) least common and most strongly condemned. The finding that only two per cent of Indian women aged between 15 and 24 years reported a non-marital partner in the past 12 months is consistent with this expectation (National AIDS Control Organisation, India and UNICEF, 2002). But even in societies where pre-marital sex is common, willingness to report may vary. In Southern Africa, for instance, where high levels of pre-marital pregnancy and HIV infections are found among young people, a huge disjuncture between publicly acclaimed sexual morality and actual behaviour engenders 'a culture of silence' on sexual matters that may well inhibit valid reporting in research studies. In much of West Africa, such considerations appear to apply with less force and honest disclosure may be more common. The implication is that inter-societal comparisons of sexual behaviour are an extremely hazardous undertaking.

Gender-related differences in reporting of sexual activity among young single survey respondents are strikingly large in most developing countries. In Latin American surveys, for instance, between 50 and 70 per cent of single men aged between 15 and 24 years report experience of heterosexual intercourse. The corresponding figures for women range from five to 25 per cent. In Asia, this gender divide is equally large and it is also apparent in some though not all African surveys. Several possible explanations have been posited but the balance of evidence strongly suggests that greater concealment of non-marital partners by women than men is the dominant cause. Biomedical validation usually shows higher sero-positivity among self-reported virgin females than males (Buvé *et al.*, 2001). HIV-positive wives comprise a larger fraction of all HIV-discordant couples than might be expected from behavioural self-reports (Allen *et al.*, 2003). Women's responses are more sensitive to mode of data collection (Gregson *et al.*, 2004). And, lastly, a unique local census of sexual partnerships in Tanzania provided rather clear-cut evidence of sex-selective under-reporting (Nnko *et al.*, 2004).

The effect of *survey design* on reporting styles is most emphatically illustrated by a comparison of two DHSs and three sexual behaviour surveys

(SBSs) in Zambia (Slaymaker and Buckner, 2004). The SBSs used a much shorter questionnaire than DHSs with a sharper focus on HIV and related behaviour. They consistently yielded much lower estimates of high-risk sexual behaviour than the two DHSs, suggesting perhaps that the longer DHS instrument allowed greater rapport to be developed before the more sensitive questions on sex were broached, than was possible in the SBSs. Even changes in the sequence or phrasing of questions can affect responses. For instance, in the late 1990s, the DHS changed its measurement of number of partners in the preceding year from a single global question to repeated strings of detailed questions about the last three partners. Comparison of results from earlier with more recent surveys shows implausibly large declines in the percentage of men who report more than one partner. The most likely explanation is that interviewers in the more recent surveys, eager to minimise repetition of sensitive questions, implicitly or perhaps explicitly, discouraged respondents from reporting more than one partner. Lastly, and not unexpectedly, certain *sexual practices* (for example, anal sex) and certain types of partner (for example, same sex) are probably more prone to concealment than other practices and partners though this tendency is difficult to verify.

This litany of problems appears to justify an unfavourable verdict on the dependability of the survey method to provide useful information on people's sexual behaviour. Indeed, it is true that abuses of survey data are more common than uses. However, repeated surveys in the same population circumvent many of these problems and there are grounds for a more positive verdict about the ability of surveys to provide valid trend data, provided that survey design is held constant. We are unaware of any population in which the incidence of HIV or other sexually transmitted infection has declined substantially without corroborative trends in behaviour. Uganda and Thailand are the two obvious examples (Nelson *et al.*, 1996; Kamali *et al.*, 2000) of such decline and corroborative trends. Of equal importance is the absence of evidence of appreciable changes in behaviour in countries with no indications, thus far, of falls in HIV incidence (Bessinger *et al.*, 2003).

Even in populations where widespread under-reporting of non-marital sex has probably occurred, repeated surveys appear to provide valid information on the direction and nature of change despite concerns that willingness to report sexual activity may change over time. Analysis of DHS data for young single women in Latin America yielded a coherent and convincing picture of change. Pre-marital sex increased, as did contraceptive use but not sufficiently to offset the protective effect of virginity with the consequence that pre-marital conceptions also increased (Ali *et al.*, 2003; Ali and Cleland, 2005). In the next section, this relative strength of the survey method is exploited to depict trends in the sexual behaviour of young people in Latin America and Africa.

Use of surveys to track trends in Latin America

In its Latin American surveys, DHS routinely collects detailed histories of contraceptive use, in the form of a month-by month calendar that covers a span of five years prior to the survey date. Interviewers are trained to enter into the calendar any births that occurred and these act as points of reference for entry of episodes of contraceptive use and any miscarriages or induced abortions that are reported (though no attempt is made to distinguish between the two). The main purpose is to allow the detailed analysis of contraceptive failure, discontinuation and switching between methods but it also provides a powerful means of monitoring trends in exposure to risks of pregnancy and infection among single women. When the date of first intercourse (ascertained earlier in the interview) is added to the calendar data, each month can be classified into the following main states: virgin, sexually active and unprotected, sexually active but protected by condoms or non-barrier contraceptive methods, and pregnant. Results can then be summarised in terms of the percentage of months (that is, time) spent in the different states. One main limitation of this classification is the lack of month-by month information on sexual behaviour. This absence makes it necessary to assume that, once sexual debut has occurred, sexual activity is regular. A second limitation is the lack of data on consistency of condom use.

Table 1.2 shows how these data can be used to track trends among never married women aged 15 to 24 for North-East Brazil, and four countries where at least two DHS surveys have been conducted. The left-hand column shows the percentage of time in the five years preceding each survey that was protected by virginity. The reported prevalence of virginity varies widely but, in each of the five settings, it has declined, most sharply in Brazil and Colombia. This trend implies that age at sexual debut has fallen. The second column shows the percentage of sexually active months that were protected by any method of contraception and the next column indicates the contribution of condoms to such protection. In the Dominican Republic, contraceptive use is low and did not change. In the other four settings, however, the percentage of months protected by contraception has increased and, again, these changes are most pronounced in Brazil and Colombia. Moreover, the share of contraceptive use represented by condoms has increased everywhere except Guatemala. In North-East Brazil, Colombia, Dominican Republic and Peru, the condom was a rarely used method in the late 1980s and early 1990s, accounting for only about 10 per cent of overall protection. By the time of the most recent survey, spanning the mid- to late-1990s, the contribution of condoms had risen to 15 per cent in the Dominican Republic and to over 20 per cent in Brazil, Colombia and Peru.

The effects of these behavioural changes on the incidence of sexually transmitted infections, including HIV, cannot be estimated because no such information was collected. However, the effect on pregnancy rates can be

Table 1.2 Trends in virginity, time protected by contraception, contribution of condoms to protection and conception rates, for Latin American population with two or more DHSs

Site/survey date	Percentage of time in last 5 years protected by virginity	Percentage of time in last 5 years sexually active but protected by contraception	Contribution of condom to protection (%)	Conception rate (per 100 woman-years)	
				All single women	Sexually active women
Brazil Northeast					
1991	82.6	27.6	10.1	3.8	26.5
1996	73.0	37.4	25.4	5.9	25.8
Colombia					
1990	80.8	21.4	6.6	3.7	22.7
1995	68.1	40.9	16.6	5.3	19.3
2000	58.2	48.6	27.4	6.2	16.7
Dominican Republic					
1991	90.8	14.8	1.8	1.1	13.0
1996	85.1	14.9	15.4	2.1	15.8
Guatemala					
1995	88.2	4.2	45.7	2.6	27.0
1998/99	83.7	10.4	32.6	4.1	31.4
Peru					
1992	80.3	21.0	8.2	3.9	23.3
1996	75.6	31.5	17.9	4.6	22.0
2002	71.7	30.9	22.1	4.9	20.2

gauged. Two types of rate are shown in Table 1.2. The first shows the rate based on all single women aged between 15 and 24 years including virgins. In all five settings, rates have increased and this trend suggests that the rise in contraceptive practice has been overshadowed by the decline in the protection of virginity. Because of the reluctance to report induced abortions, most of these pregnancies result in childbirth. Some are legitimised by shotgun weddings but the majority are born to single mothers. The right-hand column shows pregnancy rates for the sexually active only and thus permits an assessment of the impact of increased contraceptive uptake on pregnancy risk. In Colombia, where contraceptive protection increased most sharply, pregnancy rates for the sexually active have declined appreciably. Smaller declines are apparent in Brazil and Peru. In the Dominican Republic, contraceptive practice did not change and it is no surprise therefore that pregnancies became more common. In Guatemala, contraception increased slightly but nevertheless the pregnancy rate rose.

It is not claimed that the DHS data from these five surveys provide a fully accurate picture of the sexual and reproductive lives of young women in this region. On the contrary, it is likely that many sexually active women have declared themselves to be virgins and it is almost certainly true that most induced abortions have remained unreported. But the broad direction of change in these countries is plausible, coherent, internally consistent and probably valid. What appears to have happened in the 1990s is that codes of female chastity have weakened, perhaps under the influence of the more permissive values of North America and Europe, resulting in greater sexual experience before marriage. At the same time, widespread publicity about AIDS and perhaps increased access through social marketing campaigns have brought about substantial and welcome increases in condom use. Indeed, the figures in Table 1 make it clear that condoms are the only method of contraception to record a rise in use during the 1990s. This rise in condom use is starting to reduce pregnancy rates, and by implication risks of infection among the sexually active in some countries.

Tracking trends in sub-Saharan Africa

In sub-Saharan Africa, contraceptive use is generally much lower than in Latin America and so DHS enquiries rarely use the contraceptive calendar. However, information is routinely collected on age at sexual debut, number of sexual partners in the past 12 months, recency of last intercourse and whether a condom was used, and current method of contraception (if any). In a smaller number of surveys, similar information is collected from samples of men. This information is sufficient to monitor changes over time in virginity, in multiple partnerships and condom use, indicators of behaviour that correspond to the familiar three-pronged abstinence, be faithful and condom (ABC) HIV prevention strategy. However, for reasons explained in the earlier paragraph on survey design and reporting styles, it is inadvisable to use DHS to monitor trends in multiple partnerships because of major changes in the questions used to elicit this information.

In an impressive 18 African countries, trends in abstinence and condom use can be tracked for women because two or more comparable surveys have been conducted. These countries comprise 56 per cent of the total population of sub-Saharan Africa. The median date of the earliest survey round is March 1993 and, for the most recent round, June 2001, a span of a little over seven years. A convenient way to summarise trends from such a large number of surveys is to compare the pattern of results in the two survey rounds by means of pairs of box and whisker plots. The vertical length of a box indicates the values within which 50 per cent of estimates lie and the horizontal line within the box represents the median value. The vertical lines protruding from the box (the whiskers) show the values within which 95 per cent of estimates are predicted to lie. Dots outside the whiskers are extreme values.

Figures 1.1 and 1.2 show trends in sexual abstinence for never married women aged between 15 and 24 years. Two indicators of abstinence are included – no experience of sexual intercourse (or virginity) and no inter-course in the three months preceding the survey among sexually experienced women (or secondary abstinence). Interpretation of the top left-hand plot in Figure 1.1 is as follows. Among the 18 African surveys conducted around 1993, the median percentage of single women who declared themselves as virgins was about 60 per cent and, in half of these surveys, this figure lies between 50 and 80 per cent. By 2001, the median still remained at about 60 per cent but the size of the box had shrunk indi-cating a convergence in the percentage who were virgins in these 18 countries. Trends in secondary abstinence (Figure 1.2) indicate a slight increase, from a median value of 44 per cent in the earliest round to 49 per cent in the most recent round. Again the size of the box has contracted, indicating convergence in reported behaviour. The main conclusion is clear – no major changes towards greater abstinence, in response to the threat of HIV, occurred among young single women in the 1990s.

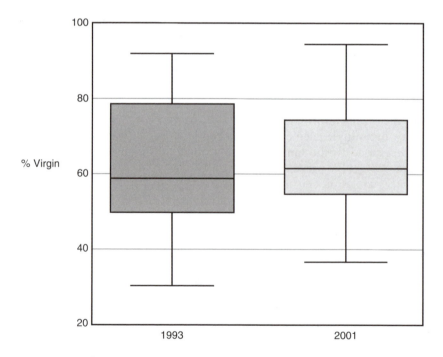

Figure 1.1 Trends (1993–2001) in standardised per cent virgin, among single women aged 15–24: 18 African countries

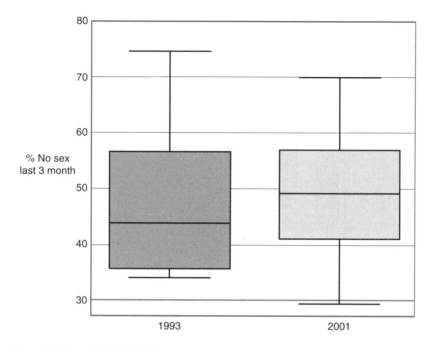

Figure 1.2 Trends (1993–2001) in standardised per cent who did not have sex in the last 3 months among sexually experienced single women aged 15–24: 18 African countries

Figure 1.3 shows trends in current use of contraceptive methods among single women who were sexually active in the past three months in the same 18 countries using the same presentational device. Current use of modern non-barrier methods (mainly oral contraceptives) changed little while use of so-called traditional methods (mainly periodic abstinence) declined. Use of condoms, however, increased from a median of about 5 to 19 per cent. By around 2001, condoms had become by far the most common method of pregnancy prevention.

More recent DHS enquiries included an additional question on use of condoms at most recent intercourse. This question was in a different section of the questionnaire from the questions on contraception and made no mention of the motive for use (pregnancy or disease prevention). Comparison of the two answers is possible in 13 of the 18 countries and provides an insight into condom use that is not primarily motivated by the desire to avoid pregnancy. In these 13 countries the median percentage reporting condom use at most recent coitus was 28 per cent. Of these 2140 women, 59 per cent had earlier said that they were currently using a condom for family planning, 7 per cent reported use of a modern non-barrier

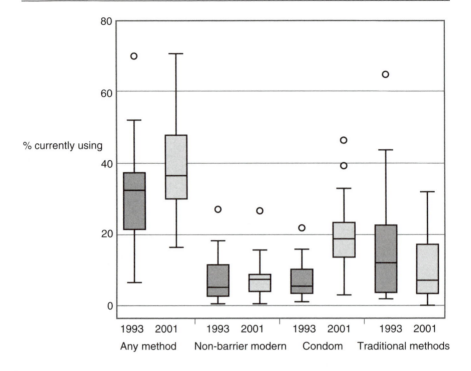

Figure 1.3 Trends (1993–2001) in current contraceptive use among single women aged 15–24 who had sex in the last 3 months: 18 African countries

method, 5 per cent were using a traditional method while the remainder (25 per cent) had declared that they were using no method. These results give rise to two important observations. First, it appears that over half of female condom users are motivated entirely or partially by the desire to avoid pregnancy. Second, double-method protection is uncommon.

Behavioural trends among young women in sub-Saharan Africa and in Latin America share one common feature; namely, increased resort to condoms. In both regions this method is becoming the dominant means of protection against unintended pregnancy with the huge added advantage of protection against infections, including HIV. However, the two regions differ with regard to trends in sexual abstinence before marriage. In Latin America, pre-marital sexual experience is increasing while in Africa there is no evidence of widespread change. This difference comes as no surprise. In Latin America, as in much of Europe, North America and Asia, high value has been placed traditionally on pre-marital chastity for women, if not for men. The apparent relaxation in codes governing sexual expression for young women in Latin America are consistent with similar well-established trends in these other regions. In most African societies, by contrast, similar value has not been placed on virginity for decades and perhaps for genera-tions. Sexual intimacy and often pregnancy and childbirth are often the pathway to the establishment of marriage and other forms of stable part-nership. Thus the liberalisation of sexual norms that have affected most regions was never likely to have the same impact in Africa as elsewhere.

Concluding comments

The central message of this chapter is that survey data on the sexual behav-iour of young people have to be handled with great caution but nevertheless have huge potential to add to an understanding of what is changing in their lives. Survey evidence can act as an invaluable corrective to the pessimistic impression often given by qualitative investigations. An aura of despon-dency and frustration hangs over the arena of HIV prevention. Despite the expenditure of huge sums of money, only two countries, Thailand and Uganda, have clearly checked their AIDS epidemics. Even well-designed and intensive interventions directed at young people have a modest record of success (Jemmott and Jemmott, 2000). Increasingly, it is argued that major transformations in gender relations or major economic improvements are essential preconditions for the desired changes in the behaviour of young men and women to take place (Kim and Watts, 2005). Men are frequently portrayed as prisoners of social constructions of masculinity that mandate sexual predation and stress the priority of immediate pleasure over longer-term health considerations, while young women are portrayed as equally imprisoned by concepts of femininity that stress passivity and acquiescence. This combination, it is argued, is disastrous for sexual health and has to be transformed before significant progress can be expected.

We do not dispute for a moment that changes toward greater gender equality are highly desirable in their own right and that poverty-reduction should be a top international priority. However, the evidence presented in this chapter provides grounds for optimism. Specifically, condom use is spreading and this could not have happened without the endorsement of men. Some will argue that the consequences of AIDS are so severe and the pace of change so modest that this optimism is unjustified. In Africa, con-dom use has increased by 1.4 per cent per annum, or 14 per cent per decade. This is approximately the same rate of change recorded for the spread of contraception in marriage in poor countries over past decades and repre-sents a much more rapid change than recorded for other health-threatening behaviours, such as cigarette smoking. Moreover, in our view it was naïve to expect abrupt changes in behaviour in response to public health messages about the dangers of sex. We suspect that AIDS-prevention messages, typi-cally constructed in the West, were initially distrusted as alien. For behaviour to change, both the nature of the problem and the solutions have to be 'domesticated' (Cleland and Watkins, 2006). This process of domestication represents the passing of ownership of the agenda from the world of international and national agencies to people themselves. It takes place through discussion and evaluation among networks of friends and relatives. This process inevitably takes time, though it can be most effectively accelerated by policies that genuinely foster local ownership. This feature may explain why Uganda was successful in containing the spread of HIV whereas Botswana failed (Allen and Heald, 2004).

The lessons about uses and abuses of surveys are also relevant to the design and evaluation of programmes for young people. Baseline survey data on the nature and magnitude of sexual and reproductive health problems should be viewed with some scepticism, assessed against all other available evidence and augmented by qualitative evidence. Endline or evaluation surveys should use an identical or very similar design to the baseline survey, in order to maximise comparability of responses. Finally, surveys should ideally be conducted by an organisation that does not have a vested interest in the success of the project, for this strategy will enhance the credibility of findings.

References

Ali, M.M., Cleland, J. and Shah, I.H. (2003) Trends in reproductive behaviour among young single women in Colombia and Peru: 1985–99, *Demography*, 40(4), 659–73.

Ali, M.M. and Cleland, J. (2005) Sexual and reproductive behaviour among single women aged 15–24 in eight Latin American countries: A comparative analysis, *Social Science and Medicine*, 60(6), 1175–85.

Allen, T. and Heald, S. (2004) HIV/AIDS policy in Africa: What has worked in Uganda and what has failed in Botswana? *Journal of International Development*, 16(8), 1141–54.

Allen, S., Meinzen-Derr, J., Kautzman, M., Zulu, I., Trask, S., Fideli, U., Musonda, R., Kasolo, F., Gao, F. and Haworth, A. (2003) Sexual behavior of HIV-discordant couples after HIV counseling and testing, *AIDS*, 17(5), 733–40.

Ankrah, E.M. (1989) AIDS: Methodological problems in studying its prevention and spread, *Social Science & Medicine*, 29(3), 265–76.

Barreto, T., Campbell, O.M. and Davies, L. (1992) Investigating induced abortion in developing countries: Methods and problems, *Studies in Family Planning*, 23, 159–70.

Bessinger, R., Akwara, P. and Halperin, D. (2003) *Sexual Behaviour, HIV and Fertility Trends: A comparative analysis of six countries*, Phase 1 of the ABC study University of North Carolina, MEASURE Evaluation Project.

Biddlecom, A. (2004) Trends in sexual behaviours and infections among young persons in the United States, *Sexually Transmitted Infections*, 80 (Suppl II), ii74–ii79.

Binson, D. and Catania, J.A. (1998) Respondents' understanding of the words used in sexual behaviour questions, *Public Opinion Quarterly*, 62, 190–208.

Blanc, A.K. and Rutenberg, N. (1991) Coitus and contraception – The utility of data on sexual intercourse for family-planning programs, *Studies in Family Planning*, 22, 162–76.

Buvé, A., Lagarde, E., Caraël, M., Rutenberg, N., Ferry, B., Glynn, F.R., Laourou, M., Akam, E., Chege, J. and Sukwa, T. for the Study Group on Heterogeneity of HIV Epidemics in African Cities (2001) Interpreting sexual behaviour data: Validity issues in the multicentre study on factors determining the differential spread of HIV in four African cities, *AIDS*, 15 (Suppl 4), S117–S126.

Cleland, J. and Ferry B. (eds) (1995) *Sexual Behaviour and AIDS in the Developing World*, London: Taylor and Francis.

Cleland, J.G., Ali, M.M. and Capo-Chichi, V. (1999) Post-partum sexual abstinence in West Africa: Implications for HIV control and family planning programme, *AIDS*, 13, 125–31.

Cleland, J., Boerma, J.T., Carael, M. and Weir, S.S. (2004) Monitoring sexual behaviour in general populations: A synthesis of lessons of the past decade, *Sexually Transmitted Infections*, 80 (Suppl 2), ii1–ii7.

Cleland, J. and Watkins, S.C. (2006) The key lesson of family planning programmes for HIV/AIDS control, *AIDS*, 20(1), 1–3.

Cowan, F.M., Langhaug, L.F., Mashungupa, G.P., Nyamurera, T., Hargrove, J., Jaffar, S., Peeling, R.W., Brown, D.W.G., Power, R., Johnson, A.M., Stephenson, J.M., Bassett, M.T. and Hayes, R.J. for the Regai Dzive Shiri Project (2002) School-based HIV prevention in Zimbabwe: Feasibility and acceptability of evaluation trials using biological outcomes, *AIDS*, 16(12), 1673–78.

Enel, C., Lagarde, E. and Pison, G. (1994) The evaluation of surveys of sexual behaviour: A study of couples in rural Senegal, *Health Transition Review*, 4 (Suppl), 111–24.

Fenton, K.A., Johnson, A.M., McManus, S. and Erens, B. (2001) Measuring sexual behaviour: Methodological challenges in survey research, *Sexually Transmitted Infections*, 77(2), 84–92.

Ferry, B., Caraël, M., Buvé, A., Auvert, B., Laourou, M., Kanhonou, L., de Loenzien, M., Akam, E., Chege, J. and Kaona, F. for the Study Group on Heterogeneity of HIV Epidemics in African Cities (2001) Comparison of key parameters of sexual behaviour in four African urban populations with different levels of HIV infection, *AIDS*, 15 (Suppl 4), S41–S50.

Frank, O. (1994) International research on sexual behaviour and reproductive health: A brief review with reference to methodology, *Annual Review of Sex Research*, 5, 1–49.

Gregson, S., Zhuwau, T., Ndlovu, J. and Nyamukapa, C.A. (2002) Methods to reduce social desirability bias in sex surveys in low-development settings: Experience from Zimbabwe, *Sexually Transmitted Diseases*, 29(10), 568–75.

Gregson, S., Mushati, P., White, P., Mlilo, M., Mundandi, C. and Myamukapa, C. (2004) Informal confidential voting interview methods and temporal changes in reported sexual risk behaviour for HIV transmission in sub-Saharan Africa, *Sexually Transmitted Infections*, 80 (Suppl II), ii36–ii42.

Hewett, P.C., Mensch, B.S. and Erulkar, A.S. (2004) Consistency in the reporting of sexual behaviour by adolescent girls in Kenya: A comparison of interviewing methods, *Sexually Transmitted Infections*, 80 (Suppl II), ii43–ii48.

Hubert, M., Bajos, N. and Sandfort, T. (1998) *Sexual Behaviour and HIV/AIDS in Europe*, London: UCL Press.

Huygens, P., Kajura, E., Seeley, J. and Barton, T. (1996) Rethinking methods for the study of sexual behaviour, *Social Science and Medicine*, 42(2), 221–31.

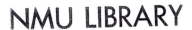

Jemmott, J.B. and Jemmott, L.S. (2000) HIV risk reduction interventions with heterosexual adolescents, *AIDS*, 14, S40–S52.

Kamali, A., Carpenter, L.M., Whitworth, J.A.G., Pool, R., Ruberantwari, A. and
Ojwiya, A. (2000) Seven-year trends in HIV-1 infection rates and changes in sexual behaviour among adults in rural Uganda, *AIDS*, 14(4), 427–34.

Kim, J.C. and Watts, C.H. (2005) Gaining a foothold: Tackling poverty, gender
inequality, and HIV in Africa, *British Medical Journal*, 331, 769–72.

Lestheaghe, R. (ed.) (1989) *Reproduction and Social Organization in Africa*,
Berkeley: University of California Press.

Malinowski, B. (1929) *The Sexual Life of Savages*, New York: Harcourt Brace
Jovanovich.

Mead, M. (1949) *Male and Females: A study of sex in a changing world*, New York:
W. Morrow.

Mensch, B.S., Hewett, P.C. and Erulkar, A.S. (2003) The reporting of sensitive
behaviour by adolescents, *Demography*, 40(2), 247–68.

National AIDS Control Organisation (India), United Nations Children's Fund
(2002) *Knowledge, Attitudes and Practices of Young Adults (15–24 years):
Disaggregated data from the National Behavioural Surveillance Survey (2001)*,
New Delhi: NACO and UNICEF.

Nelson, K.E., Celentano, D.D., Eiumtrakol, S., Hoover, D.R., Beyrer, C., Suprasert,
S., Kuntolbutra, S. and Khamboonruang, C. (1996) Changes in sexual behaviour
and decline in HIV infection among young men in Thailand, *New England
Journal of Medicine*, 335, 297–303.

Nnko, S., Boerma, J.T., Urassa, M., Mwaluko, G. and Zaba, B. (2004) Secretive
females or swaggering males? An assessment of the quality of sexual partnership
reporting in rural Tanzania, *Social Science and Medicine*, 59(2), 299–310.

Obeymeyer, C.M. (2005) Reframing research on sexual behaviour and HIV, *Studies
in Family Planning*, 36(1), 1–12.

Plummer, M.L., Ross, D.A., Wight, D., Changalucha, J., Mshana, G., Wamoyi, J.,
Todd, J., Anemone, A., Mosha, F.F., Obasi, A.I.N. and Hayes, R.J. (2004) 'A bit
more truthful': The validity of adolescent sexual behaviour data collected in rural
northern Tanzania using five methods, *Sexually Transmitted Infections*, 80
(Suppl II), ii49–ii56.

Schenk, K. and Williamson, J. (2005) Ethical approaches to gathering information
from children and adolescents in international settings: Guidelines and resources,
Washington, DC: Population Council.

Slaymaker, E. and Zaba, B. (2003) Measurement of condom use as a risk factor for
HIV infection, *Reproductive Health Matters*, 11(22), 174–84.

Slaymaker, E. and Buckner B. (2004) Monitoring trends in sexual behaviour in
Zambia, 1996–2003, *Sexually Transmitted Infections*, 80 (Suppl II), ii85–ii90.

Weinhardt, L.S., Forsyth, A.D., Carey, M.P., Jaworski, B.D. and Durant, L.E. (1998)
Reliability and validity of self-report measures of HIV-related sexual behavior:
Progress since 1990 and recommendations for research and practice, *Archives of
Sexual Behavior*, 27(2), 155–80.

Westoff, C. (1974) Coital frequency and contraception, *Family Planning
Perspectives*, 6, 136–41.

Chapter 2

Young people and condom use

Findings from qualitative research

Cicely Marston, Eleanor King and Roger Ingham

Introduction

There is a range of methods appropriate to the study of sexual activity amongst young people, and each has particular strengths and weaknesses; whichever method or combination of methods is selected depends on what is being explored, and why. To take a simple example, while a survey might be designed to answer questions such as 'what percentage of young people report use of a condom at their most recent sexual intercourse', a qualitative study, through asking more open (and normally in-depth) questions, would attempt to delve more fully into the range of reasons why condoms are, or are not, used on particular occasions and with particular people.

When well designed and rigorously used, qualitative approaches take account of the fact that sexual behaviour is highly complex. They can be used for various purposes, including description, explanation and the development of new concepts and theories. They have the potential, when used appropriately, to unravel some of the complexities involved in all aspects of sexual behaviour. As such, qualitative studies can stand alone, or complement quantitative approaches, such as those drawn upon in Ali and Cleland's chapter in this volume.

Qualitative methods are able to capture complexity and diversity in ways that quantitative approaches simply cannot achieve. The box below contains some of the questions typically asked in surveys about condom use. Responses are limited to the options available, and other possible answers cannot be considered.

In qualitative work, on the other hand, participants use their own words, ideas and phrasing to address issues. Producing detailed descriptions, however, may not be the only goal of qualitative studies. As with most research, the ultimate contribution of many studies using qualitative methods is towards the development of general theory – that is, theory which has relevance beyond the circumstances of each specific study. While descriptive accounts of diversity, change over time, and so on, can be valuable – for instance, to assess local needs for programmes and services, or to identify

---

1 Uganda DHS women's questionnaire (response options shown in parentheses)

The last time you had sexual intercourse, was a condom used? (yes; no)
What was the main reason you used a condom on that occasion? (respondent wanted to prevent STD/HIV; respondent wanted to prevent pregnancy; respondent wanted to prevent both STD/HIV and pregnancy; did not trust partners/feels partner has other partners; partner insisted; other; don't know)
What was the main reason for not using a condom? (respondent wanted to become pregnant; trusted partner; partner insisted; other; don't know)

Source: Uganda Bureau of Statistics and ORC Macro (2001)

2 Australian survey of men's condom use (all yes–no responses)

Have you ever used condoms to have sex with a woman?
Have you used condoms in the last six months to have sex with a woman?
During the past six months, how often did you have vaginal intercourse with your partner where you ejaculated inside her?
When you did this, how often was a condom used?
The last time you had sex [with a woman], did you put your penis into her vagina?
Was a condom used?
Was the condom put on before your penis touched her vagina?

Source: De Visser et al. (2003)

---

new statistical associations with other variables – general theories which can be used to understand behaviour in numerous places at different time periods are more powerful tools. Many individual studies are not explicitly theoretical, yet they may nevertheless be able to provide valuable insights that can be used to improve theoretical understanding. A theory, once postulated, can then be adapted, supported or rejected as new evidence comes to light.

The qualitative methods available to investigate young people's sexual health include unstructured or, more commonly, semi-structured interviews (sometimes referred to as individual depth interviews) and focus group discussions, as well as, less commonly, text analysis (for example, media analysis) observation and ethnography. The choice of methods depends on the type of information that is sought. For instance, to elicit sensitive information about a young person's own sexual experiences, a one-on-one interview might be preferred. On the other hand, to study how young people speak to each other about 'virginity', or social norms regarding gender relations, for example, a focus group discussion might be a more appropriate method. Whether the group is formed from people who already know one another, or strangers, or whether it is composed of young people of the same sex or a mixture, will also depend on what the researcher hopes to find out. The researcher might choose single-sex groups, for example, to examine how particular topics are discussed in such environments, or perhaps to encourage free speech if discussions are to cover aspects of sexual behaviour not usually broached in mixed-sex groups.

It is important to note, however, that, although single-sex focus groups are common, they are not obligatory. Men and women have been observed to use distinct vocabularies and styles of speech (Marston, 2004), and analysis of conversation in single-sex groups must take this into account. Similarly, a mixed-sex group may be selected deliberately to explore gender relations and styles of communication between the sexes. To observe how young people speak and act in more natural settings, participant observation can be used.

In more thorough studies – and where funding allows – researchers may attempt to obtain data using a variety of sources and methods to allow comparison between them, and to increase the reliability of the conclusions reached (for example, Middelthon, 2001). There are no fixed rules about how this should be done; researchers from different disciplinary backgrounds favour different combinations of methods, with anthropologists, for example, traditionally using participant observation and unstructured interviews as their key methods. In recent multi-disciplinary literature on young people's sexual behaviour, however, anthropological approaches are less commonly seen (exceptions include Wight, 1994); more frequent are focus group or other interview methods with no participant observation component.

Analysis of qualitative data usually involves researchers identifying themes and topics that emerge from the interviews or other data collection methods. These themes and topics may then be explored further in subsequent data collection. The analytical process is iterative; the themes identified in the first round of analysis are refined in a second round, and can change to take account of new findings that emerge and any new insights that are gained. The themes identified after several rounds of analysis should form a robust and increasingly theoretical reflection of the content of the data analysed. Many textbooks are available for consultation on qualitative methods, analysis and theory (for example, Hammersley, 1998; Wetherell et al., 2001; Green and Browne, 2005).

One clear advantage of qualitative methods is that they allow non-researchers, in this case young people, to have a say about what they think, feel and know. Qualitative studies can allow a detailed exploration of people's stated motives, their social environments, their understanding of particular concepts, the wide range of meanings that are attached to specific activities or objects, and other important aspects of their lives. In return for the depth achieved in many of these studies, however, there is often a corresponding lack of breadth; it is very difficult, for example, to interview in depth every type of person in a population who might use a condom. It is essential to make up for the inevitable lack of breadth by ensuring that the study has genuine depth. Qualitative studies usually concentrate on particular groups of interest; for example, young people living in low-income areas of Mexico City (Marston, 2005). One major advantage of qualitative approaches lies in their ability to suggest new theoretical ways to understand behaviour which may, or may not, apply beyond the specific groups studied. If the work is done in a superficial way, for example, where analysis is shallow, or where questions have been used that are more suited to survey-type research, the study risks both failing to achieve the depth of a good qualitative study, and simultaneously suffering lack of breadth.

Distinguishing between good and bad qualitative studies is obviously important. There are no set definitions of what makes a study 'good' but, in one large-scale literature review carried out by the first two authors of this chapter (Marston and King, 2006), studies of young people's sexual behaviour were classified into high-quality and low-quality studies. The high-quality studies had to contain either a detailed description, or be theory-building. Their conclusions also had to be based on empirical evidence. Low-quality studies lacked these features. Despite this rather generous definition of high quality, most studies failed to meet these requirements. Low-quality studies, on the other hand, were abundant. For instance, there were numerous low-quality studies that attempted to explain use or non-use of condoms, but which only described focus group discussions of young men's attitudes to condom use. The write-ups usually provided an uncritical report of what the men said, without taking into account the fact that the focus group situation itself might have affected what they were prepared to say, or the fact that general opinions about liking or disliking condoms may not translate into practice. Because the studies lacked depth, they simply serve as a record of what the particular men in those particular focus groups said at that time – they do not provide any deeper insight that might be applicable more generally. On the other hand, higher quality studies (such as Holland *et al.*, 1998) take account of the contextual factors affecting both behaviour and what interviewees are likely to say in particular circumstances. They are also more reflexive, that is, the researchers take account of the effects they themselves have on the research process (for example, see Wight, 1994).

Qualitative research into young people's sexual behaviour is increasingly popular because of the strengths of qualitative methods described above. Sexual behaviours, like any social behaviours, are highly diverse. Individuals, themselves diverse, interact in a variety of different social and cultural contexts. Some young men and women are sexually active, others are not; some engage in sexual activity with members of the opposite sex, some with same-sex partners, some are coerced into sex, some desire it, some are encouraged to engage in sexual activity, and some are prohibited. For each individual, these factors change over time and across different stages in the life course. In any social setting there is therefore a great diversity of possible experiences and behaviours, depending on individual personalities and attributes, family structures, social expectations, and many other factors.

Very few studies of young people's sexual behaviour were carried out before 1990 but, since then, and in the shadow of the global HIV pandemic, there has been a dramatic increase in the quantity of studies, the topics that they focus upon, and the areas of the world in which they have been carried out. Qualitative work has enabled insights to be gained into the social and cultural processes affecting various aspects of sexual activity; in the remainder of this chapter we provide a brief overview of some of the results from such studies; one seemingly simple behaviour – whether or not condoms are used – is used as an example to illustrate some of the ways in which qualitative methods have been valuable in providing insight into the real complexities involved in this action.

Although these open-ended approaches are ideal for exploring in detail the impact of different social and cultural contexts, this specific example reveals some fairly consistent patterns across a range of different settings.

The condom: more than just a physical device

Use or non-use of condoms has been of particular interest to public health researchers trying to describe young people's sexual behaviour. Condoms are of clinical interest because of their dual role in protecting against pregnancy whilst simultaneously reducing the risk of transmission of sexually transmitted infections, including HIV. The symbolic and social significance of condoms and their use, however, has often been ignored by public health specialists and some HIV prevention workers.

Young people who only sometimes use condoms for sexual intercourse outside marriage (or with non-marital partners), are simply characterised as 'inconsistent' in many survey reports (for example, Pettifor et al., 2005), and campaigns to encourage young people to use condoms have often assumed that ignorance or non-availability are the main reasons for non-use. However, it has become increasingly evident both that 'inconsistency' can be misleading as an explanation of young people's behaviour (see below), and that making a young person aware that condoms can protect against pregnancy and disease does not guarantee that he or she will go on to use them; the link between knowledge of condoms and their use is far from clear (for example, see Sheeran et al., 1999; Marston et al., 2004).

Qualitative research has begun to illuminate this area and explain why apparent discrepancies arise. Key areas in terms of condom use that have been identified include perceptions about the 'riskiness' of a particular partner (or category of partners), the symbolic significance of condoms and their use, and the interactional power dynamics that can affect the likelihood of use. Similar factors have also been found to be important in understanding other aspects of sexual activity but, for the sake of simplicity, only condom use is discussed here.

Risk perception: clean and unclean partners

One near-universal finding is that young people assess the likelihood that their partners are carrying disease and are often more prepared to use condoms if they believe their partner is, in some sense, 'risky'. The disease status of the partner, however, is not usually assessed on the basis of factual information such as clinical test results. Rather, it is often based on factors such as appearance, social position, or social proximity.

In one study with South African street youth, focus group participants claimed they could assess whether or not someone was infected with HIV based on their appearance. Their descriptions included 'looking like a leper, losing one's hair, bleeding and paralysis' (Swart-Kruger and Richter, 1997: 959).

In Australia, as well as general ideas about appearance, young men made a distinction between known and unknown women in terms of perceived riskiness and need for condom use, with known women being seen less risky: '... for the guys, if it's a girl outside that [friendship] circle then yeah, condoms are used' (Waldby et al., 1993: 36).

Many young people who insist on using condoms with partners they see as risky may nevertheless refrain from using them with partners they consider to be safe. For instance, they might never use condoms with long-term girlfriends or boyfriends, but use them every time with recent or non-formal partners. This is the type of behaviour that can be typified as 'inconsistent condom use' by those whose interest is in simply describing patterns of condom use, rather than in the types of relationships in which condoms are used. It is now evident that types of partner and relationships are crucial in helping to understand whether or not condoms are used, and in helping to explain the apparent inconsistencies in usage by particular individuals. A relatively early study in the UK found that simply 'knowing' one's partner (through having attended the same school, living in the same neighbourhood, knowing that they came from a 'decent' family, or simply having 'seen them around') was sufficient justification for believing that they were safe from disease, and therefore that it was not essential to insist on condom use (Woodcock et al., 1992).

For many reasons, including perceived riskiness of the partner, and symbolic aspects of condom use (see below), it is now clear that the relationship between individuals involved in a sexual event is crucial. Type of relationship is a key predictor of condom use or non-use. Young people all over the world report enthusiasm for condoms in short-term, unstable relationships, while avoiding them for sex with girlfriends/boyfriends; this has been reported for instance in countries as diverse as the USA (Lear, 1995;

Foreman, 2003; Champion *et al.*, 2004), Thailand (Morrison, 2004), South Africa (Harrison *et al.*, 2001), Nigeria (Jordan Smith, 2004) and Nicaragua (Kalk *et al.*, 2001) among many others. This feature of condom use was initially clarified through the use of qualitative research methods; as a result, it is now also taken into account in some surveys; many now not only ask whether or not condoms were used with a particular partner, but also what the relationship was with that partner (although many surveys restrict this enquiry to a simple 'casual' versus 'steady' dichotomy which can oversimplify the real-life situation).

Assessing risk, however, may not lead to protective behaviour. The fact that a particular sexual behaviour is seen as risky can in some cases increase its desirability. In other words, the fact of knowing that it is risky can enhance its appeal rather than encourage safer behaviours, as reported for instance in Thailand (Belk *et al.*, 1998), Sweden (Christianson *et al.*, 2003) and the USA (Seal *et al.*, 2000). Sex without a condom, then, can be desired for its own sake in part because of its associations with danger.

Symbolic aspects of condom use and condoms

Perceived riskiness of the partner is only one part of the picture. In common with other sexual practices, condom use also has important symbolic dimensions. In other words, using a condom is not a simple physical act – it also has social meaning. Having sexual intercourse without a condom is often reported to be a sign of trust (Lear, 1996; Hillier *et al.*, 1999; Castaneda *et al.*, 2001). In a Norwegian study of men having sex with men, one young man commented: 'If you are in a relationship and stop using condoms, it is a confirmation of the relationship – that you treasure what is between you ...' or, as another man in the same study put it, 'If I ask him to use a condom it is as if I do not trust him' (Middelthon, 2001: 71).

In addition, fear of losing an erection has been reported as a reason for avoiding condom use in many settings. One likely reason that this fear has such a powerful effect is that maintaining an erection is bound up with ideas about masculinity – to lose an erection is seen as a symbol of not being a 'real' man (Middelthon and Aggleton, 2001).

The condom by itself, separate from the physical act of its use, has further symbolic aspects. In many places, carrying a condom can imply sexual experience with the result that women are reluctant to do so – see, for example, research in Nigeria (Jordan Smith, 2004), in Mexico (Castaneda *et al.*, 2001), in the UK (Holland *et al.*, 1998), and in Ghana (Ankomah, 1998). After a discussion of women carrying condoms, one boy in a Brazilian focus group summarised his views as follows, 'The deal is this – if she asks that we use [a condom], we will do it, but if she has it in her pocketbook, it makes her into a slut' (Levinson *et al.*, 2004: 217).

There is clearly an important relationship in this instance between the symbolism of the condom and the overarching gender stereotypes in particular communities. In a place where the sexual experience of women is less stigmatised, it would be expected that more women would be prepared to carry condoms. Conversely, and again relating to gender stereotypes, carrying a condom might be desirable for a man who wishes to imply or display his sexual activity to his peers, as reported for some young men in the UK (Holland *et al.*, 1998).

One of the consequences of these attitudes is that it can be difficult to access contraception, as this young, unmarried, Nicaraguan woman explained:

> That is why many girls do not go to the pharmacy and say 'I want to have a package of contraceptives'. Maybe there are three ladies there and they will say '... she is only 15 years old running around buying contraceptives, that is a barbarity, she must be a prostitute ...'. On the other hand, it is the other way around when a man goes to the pharmacy to buy condoms. Nobody says it is barbaric. He is only buying condoms because he has a lot of women ... Yes, there are contraceptives and they are very cheap, but a lot of people feel shame and are embarrassed to say that they want to buy contraceptives.
>
> (Berglund *et al.*, 1997: 9)

Condoms can be associated strongly with disease and immorality (Varga, 1997). In one study, a young, South African man said: 'If you wear [a condom] you appear to have AIDS, because there is no need to use a condom if you behave correctly' (Swart-Kruger and Richter, 1997: 962). Members of a focus group in Zimbabwe described what happened in a lesson where the teacher was promoting abstinence from sexual intercourse: 'one girl asked about condoms, and the teacher was very angry. She said they were dirty and that only prostitutes used them' (Marindo, 2003: 19).

Many studies have noted that associations with disease can make it difficult for some young people to request condom use. One woman in the UK reported that she and a friend used a particular strategy to circumvent this problem: 'Rather than saying "will you wear something, because I don't want to get AIDS?" which sounds really bad, doesn't it, we would say "you'll have to wear something because I'm not on the pill"' (Holland *et al.*, 1991: 137).

Condoms do not only have negative connotations, of course. Their future use can be mooted as a way of broaching the subject of sexual intercourse. One young Norwegian gay man said he used a request for condoms as an indirect way to find out whether a partner wished to engage in anal sex:

I asked if I should go and get a condom. That is how I do it. He said 'not now' and then I didn't dare to take it up again afterwards. You check out about anal intercourse through asking if you should get a condom. I use it as a sign. It is much easier than asking directly.

(Middelthon, 2001: 62)

Similarly, in the UK, one man described his condom use as follows:

I was not scared that she would have the virus. I think at the back of my mind [was] that once I pulled my condom out then that meant that I was having sex ... As opposed to ... fumbling and making a mess of it and then her changing her mind.

(Wight, 1999: 753)

In these cases, condoms were used to establish consent to intercourse, and in addition, the intent to use a condom was made clear before intercourse began.

Power

A crucial aspect of sexual relationships is the power dynamic between the couple involved, as well as with others, such as family members or peers, who might wish to influence the process of a particular relationship. A young person could decide that his or her partner was risky, could determine the need to use a condom, be prepared to carry a condom and attempt to use it, but still be unable to because the partner does not agree, for instance. The power dimension of condom use has attracted a great deal of attention in the field of health promotion, especially with respect to the relationship between power and gender.

Work in South Africa in particular has shown very clearly that violence and coercion perpetrated by men on their female partners are an integral part of sexual intercourse for many people in that setting. Women, for instance, often report that they are unable to refuse sex with boyfriends for fear of the violent consequences (Wood *et al.*, 1998 and see Chapter 7).

Much of the commentary in the public health sphere about power with respect to condom use has focused only on somewhat simplistic models of gender/power relationships. Extrapolating from findings such as those from South Africa described above, it is often assumed, for example, that gender/power structures mean that all women are necessarily disadvantaged compared with men. While it is clearly the case that many heterosexual pairings fit this model, the idea that women in general, or young women in particular, are *en masse* disempowered in sexual relationships is an oversimplification. Related assumptions permeate the public health literature. One example is that many sex education programmes take for granted that women need to be taught to 'negotiate' condom use. The reasons for this are not usually made explicit, but they appear to be related to an assumption that, in general, women want to use condoms, but men do not. There is also a secondary assumption that men will have the advantage in this type of scenario. Again, it is possible that for many couples these assumptions are justified. Nevertheless, these over-simplistic models of power relations cannot account for other key variables such as the power that may be associated with economic wealth, or with age, ethnicity, class or caste (see, for example, Hennink *et al.*, 1999; Middelthon and Aggleton, 2001), which may also play an important role, or indeed that women might also sometimes refuse to use condoms (see Chapter 4 by Ricardo *et al.* in this volume for a more detailed discussion of gender issues).

When sex takes place as part of an exchange for money or gifts, it may be particularly difficult to control whether or not condoms are used (Ankomah, 1998; Bloor *et al.*, 1990). Transactional sex is common in many parts of the world, outside the context of formal sex work, and frequently involves young people (see Chapter 8 by Busza in this volume).

When the complexities of partner relationships and the symbolic values of condoms are taken into account, the reasons for apparently paradoxical behaviour become clearer. For example, in one study in Australia, injecting drug users were extremely careful to use only clean injecting equipment, while simultaneously engaging in unprotected sex with potentially HIV-infected partners (Hillier *et al.*, 1999). Such behaviour is confusing if it is assumed that people act in order to optimise their physical health. The rationale for such behaviours is less difficult to identify once other desires are accounted for, such as maintaining or achieving emotional intimacy with a partner, which may be prioritised over condom use. It is very clear from all of the qualitative literature that young people do not necessarily focus on public health priorities when engaging in sexual activities.

Discussion

Throughout this chapter, we have focused on one apparently simple aspect of sexual behaviour – condom use – and have shown, albeit briefly, the importance of understanding its symbolic and contextual aspects. Sexual behaviour does not occur in isolation; it happens within the contexts of individuals' wider lives and experiences. To understand sexuality and sexual practices, it is vital that these contextual dimensions are taken fully into account.

Given the crucial symbolic dimensions of condom use and of sexual behaviour in general, it is not surprising that practices and accepted behaviours vary from group to group. Not only do variations exist between sub-cultures and sub-groups, but changes occur over time, perhaps in response to specific external factors. In the case of condoms, their use and even the discussion of their use has changed dramatically in response to HIV/AIDS in various countries, including Thailand (Morrison, 2004).

Despite the complexity and the diversity of behaviours within and across societies, there appear to be some core social factors affecting sexual behaviour in general, and condom use in particular, that can be identified from the research literature. These core factors allow us to begin to construct a theoretical basis for understanding of sexual behaviour in general.

Well-designed qualitative studies help to document and begin to explain the complexity of sexual behaviour, including the interplay between individual characteristics, social dynamics, and sub-cultures in which behaviours occur. It should be clear from this chapter that even something as apparently simple as condom use is a complex phenomenon. Designing a programme to meet the frequently-cited public health goal of 'increasing condom use' in different settings is therefore less straightforward than it might at first appear.

From the qualitative research literature, however, we can begin to form ideas about what might be of theoretical importance to examine when designing research to inform programmes. For instance, what are the social expectations of male and female sexual behaviour in the community where the programme will be implemented? Are there specific power dynamics associated with gender or other factors that must be taken into account? What symbolic dimensions do condoms have in the particular setting? How are risks prioritised? Of course, this should not be considered an exhaustive list, but ignoring these aspects would be ill-advised, given the findings from the studies outlined here. In this way, complexities uncovered in the individual studies can begin to contribute to a more general theoretical model, in which central concepts such as gender relations, risk perception and symbolism are linked to behaviour. The more work that is done, then the more refined these central concepts can become; some may even be rejected in time, in favour of other, more sophisticated versions as new findings come to light. From these central concepts, research can be designed to explore and describe the specific circumstances in a given setting so that programmes can take account of, and address, local diversity.

This chapter has only been able to provide an introduction to some of the possibilities of qualitative research, and the crucial role it has to play both in understanding sexual behaviour, and in designing programmes aimed at improving health. In selecting condom use as an example and showing some of its complexities, we hope to have demonstrated both the utility of qualitative research approaches, and the need to avoid taking even apparently straightforward behaviours for granted. Previously, public health opinion held that using condoms was a simple and rational response to the risk of HIV transmission through sexual intercourse. Qualitative research has revealed this to be a fallacy. Even now, some commentators view condom use as a straightforward, rational act, and do not consider the possibility that individuals' circumstances might change their desire or ability to use condoms at a given time or place. To understand the complexities of behaviour, and to design more effective sexual health programmes, contextual factors such as those described in this chapter need to be taken into account. Qualitative research has a vital role to play in this process.

References

Ankomah, A. (1998) Condom use in sexual exchange relationships among young single adults in Ghana, *AIDS Education and Prevention*, 10, 303–16.

Belk, R.W., Ostergaard, P. and Groves, R. (1998) Sexual consumption in the time of AIDS: A study of prostitute patronage in Thailand, *Journal of Public Policy and Marketing*, 17, 197–214.

Berglund, S., Liljestrand, J., De Maria Marin, F., Salgado, N. and Zelaya, E. (1997) The background of adolescent pregnancies in Nicaragua: A qualitative approach, *Social Science and Medicine*, 44, 1–12.

Bloor, M., McKeganey, N. and Barnard, M. (1990) An ethnographic study of HIV-related risk practices among Glasgow rent boys and their clients: Report of a pilot study, *AIDS Care*, 2, 17–24.

Castaneda, X.B., Brindis, C. and Camey, I.C. (2001) Nebulous margins: Sexuality and social constructions of risks in rural areas of Central Mexico, *Culture, Health and Sexuality*, 3(2), 203–19.

Champion, J.D., Shain, R.N. and Piper, J. (2004) Minority adolescent women with sexually transmitted diseases and a history of sexual or physical abuse, *Issues in Mental Health Nursing*, 25, 293–316.

Christianson, M., Johansson, E., Emmelin, M. and Westman, G. (2003) 'One-night stands' – risky trips between lust and trust: Qualitative interviews with Chlamydia trachomatis infected youth in north Sweden, *Scandinavian Journal of Public Health*, 31, 44–50.

De Visser, R.O., Smith, A.M.A., Rissel, C.E., Richters, J. and Grulich, A.E. (2003) Safer sex and condom use among a representative sample of adults, *Australian and New Zealand Journal of Public Health*, 27, 223–9.

Foreman, F.E. (2003) African American college women: Constructing a hierarchy of sexual arrangements, *AIDS Care*, 15, 493–504.

Green, J. and Browne, J. (2005) *Principles of Social Research*, Maidenhead UK: Open University Press.

Hammersley, M. (1998) *Reading Ethnographic Research: A critical guide*, London: Longman.

Harrison, A., Xaba, N. and Kunene, P. (2001) Understanding safe sex: Gender narratives of HIV and pregnancy prevention by rural South African school-going youth, *Reproductive Health Matters*, 9, 63–71.

Hennink, M., Diamond, I. and Cooper, P. (1999) Young Asian women and relationships: Traditional or transitional? *Ethnic and Racial Studies*, 22, 867–91.

Hillier, L., Dempsey, D. and Harrison, L. (1999) 'I'd never share a needle' – [but I often have unsafe sex]: Considering the paradox of young people's sex and drugs talk, *Culture, Health and Sexuality*, 1, 347–61.

Holland, J., Ramazanoglu, C., Scott, S., Sharpe, S. and Thomson, R. (1991) Between embarrassment and trust: Young women and the diversity of condom use in P. Aggleton, in G. Hart and P. Davies (eds) *AIDS: Responses, Interventions and Care*, London: Falmer Press, 127–48.

Holland, J., Ramazanoglu, C., Sharpe, S. and Thomson, R. (1998) *The Male in the Head: Young people, heterosexuality and power,* London: Tufnell Press.

Jordan Smith, D. (2004) Youth, sin and sex in Nigeria: Christianity and HIV/AIDS-related beliefs and behaviour among rural-urban migrants, *Culture, Health and Sexuality,* 6, 425–37.

Kalk, A.K., Kroeger, A., Meyer, R., Cuan, M. and Dickson, R (2001) Influences on condom use among young men in Managua, Nicaragua, *Culture, Health and Sexuality,* 3(4), 469–81.

Lear, D. (1995) Sexual communication in the age of AIDS: The construction of risk and trust among young adults, *Social Science and Medicine,* 41, 1311–23.

Lear, D. (1996) 'You're gonna be naked anyway': College students negotiating safer sex, *Qualitative Health Research,* 6, 112–34.

Levinson, R.A., Sadigursky, C. and Erchak, G.M. (2004) The impact of cultural context on Brazilian adolescents' sexual practices, *Adolescence,* 39, 203–27.

Marindo, R. (2003) Condom use and abstinence among unmarried young people in Zimbabwe: Which strategy, whose agenda? *Population Council Working Paper No. 170,* New York: Population Council.

Marston, C. (2004) Gendered communication among young people in Mexico: Implications for sexual health interventions, *Social Science and Medicine,* 59, 445–56.

Marston, C. (2005) What is heterosexual coercion? Interpreting narratives from young people in Mexico City, *Sociology of Health and Illness,* 27, 68–91.

Marston, C. and King, E. (2006, in press) Seven factors that shape young people's sexual behaviour: findings from a systematic review and comparative thematic analysis of qualitiative studies, *Lancet,* 368.

Marston, C.A., Juarez, F. and Izazola, J.A. (2004) Young unmarried men and sex: Do friends and partners shape risk behaviour? *Culture, Health and Sexuality,* 6(5), 411–24.

Middelthon, A.L. (2001) Interpretations of condom use and non-use among young Norwegian gay men: A qualitative study, *Medical Anthropology Quarterly,* 15, 58–83.

Middelthon, A.L. and Aggleton, P. (2001) Reflection and dialogue for HIV prevention among young gay men, *AIDS Care,* 13, 515–26.

Morrison, L. (2004) Traditions in transition: Young people's risk for HIV in Chiang Mai, Thailand, *Qualitative Health Research,* 14, 328–44.

Pettifor, A.E., Rees, H.V., Kleinschmidt, I., Steffenson, A.E., MacPhail, C., Hlongwa-Madikizela, L., Vermaak, K. and Padian, N.S. (2005) Young people's sexual health in South Africa: HIV prevalence and sexual behaviors from a nationally representative household survey, *AIDS,* 19, 1525–34.

Seal, D.W., Kelly, J.A., Bloom, F.R., Stevenson, L.Y., Coley, B.I. and Broyles, L.A. (2000) HIV prevention with young men who have sex with men: What young men themselves say is needed. Medical College of Wisconsin CITY Project Research Team, *AIDS Care,* 12, 5–26.

Sheeran, P., Abraham, C. and Orbell, S. (1999) Psychosocial correlates of heterosexual condom use: A meta-analysis, *Psychological Bulletin,* 125, 90–132.

Swart-Kruger, J. and Richter, L.M. (1997) AIDS-related knowledge, attitudes and behaviour among South African street youth: Reflections on power, sexuality and the autonomous self, *Social Science and Medicine,* 45, 957–66.

Uganda Bureau of Statistics and ORC Macro (2001) *Uganda Demographic and Health Survey 2000–2001*, Calverton, Maryland: UBOS and ORC Macro.

Varga, C.A. (1997) Sexual decision-making and negotiation in the midst of AIDS: Youth in KwaZulu-Natal, South Africa, *Health Transition Review*, 7, 45–67.

Waldby, C., Kippax, S. and Crawford, J. (1993) Cordon Sanitaire: 'Clean' and 'unclean' women in the AIDS discourse of young heterosexual men, in P. Aggleton, P. Davies and G. Hart (eds) *AIDS: Facing the Second Decade*, London: Falmer Press, 29–39.

Wetherell, M., Taylor, S. and Yates, S.J. (2001) *Discourse Theory and Practice*, London: Sage.

Wight, D. (1994) Boys' thoughts and talk about sex in a working-class locality of Glasgow, *Sociological Review*, 42, 703–37.

Wight, D. (1999) Cultural factors in young heterosexual men's perception of HIV risk, *Sociology of Health and Illness*, 21, 735–58.

Wood, K., Maforah, F. and Jewkes, R. (1998) 'He forced me to love him': Putting violence on adolescent sexual health agendas, *Social Science and Medicine*, 47, 233–42.

Woodcock, A., Stenner, K. and Ingham, R. (1992) Young people talking about HIV and AIDS: Interpretations of personal risk of infection, *Health Education Research: Theory and Practice*, 7(2), 229–47.

Chapter 3

The importance of context in understanding and seeking to promote sexual health

Roger Ingham

Introduction

It is commonplace to read or hear that, in order better to understand young people's sexual and reproductive behaviour and health, we need to take account of the wider contexts in which they live and act. This chapter discusses some of the meanings of the term 'context', and what might be covered in such an approach, suggests some reasons why consideration and understanding of contexts is important, explores some of the difficulties in establishing 'what works' in relation to contexts and HIV prevention, discusses some problems in 'measuring' contexts and suggests some ways forward in developing a context-based research and programmatic agenda.

What do we mean by context?

There is a long history of debate within social sciences regarding the extent to which variations in behaviour can better be understood in terms of individual characteristics – such as personality, attitudes, knowledge, and so on – or the social milieu(x) in which people live. Most people accept that both approaches have value but differ in the extent to which they orientate towards one or the other in their models and explanations; generally, psychologists emphasise the former approach, whilst sociologists and anthropologists emphasise the latter.

In the early days of increased interest in sexual activity and risk, much emphasis was placed on the use of self-completion questionnaires that attempted to 'measure' knowledge and/or awareness of HIV and routes of transmission (for example, Cleland and Ferry, 1995). Other researchers and programme developers used existing models drawn from social or health psychology – for example, the Health Belief Model (Rosenstock *et al.*, 1988), the Theory of Reasoned Action (TRA – Fishbein and Ajzen, 1975), and the Theory of Planned Behaviour (Ajzen and Madden, 1986). These use a range of dimensions, depending on the particular model, and attempt to explain the adoption of (or at least the intention to adopt) safer behaviours (for example, condom use and other means of reducing risk) in terms of the 'level' to which a variable is or is not present; the box below provides an example of the use of the TRA. Apart from the TRA, other dimensions used in a range of models include perceived vulnerability, the costs and benefits of particular courses of action, perceived severity, self-efficacy, perceived behavioural control, and others.

Although such individualistic models have guided a great deal of research into health-related behaviours, and have had some limited success in accounting for variance in behaviour (normally reported condom use in the case of sexual activity studies – see, for example, Norman and Conner, 1995 and Sheeran *et al.*, 1999), there is increasing recognition of their shortcomings, both methodologically and theoretically, as well as with respect to their contribution to programme development. For example, such models downplay the importance of factors such as commitment to work with young people on the part of political and religious leaders and/or the availability of supplies and resources such as condoms, factors that are central to young people's ability to protect themselves against unwanted sexual health outcomes such as pregnancy and sexually transmitted infections. Yet, commitment and access to services have been, for some time, well recognised internationally as essential elements of any coherent sexual health programme (UNAIDS, 1999; Makinwa and O'Grady, 2001).

Although the primary aim of this chapter is not to engage in a detailed critique of such approaches, a few points are, however, worth noting. Drawing on the work of Kippax and Crawford (1993), Ingham *et al.* (1992), Ingham (1994) and Ingham and van Zessen (1997), the following general criticisms can be made.

First, many of these theoretical frameworks are based on an assumption of individual rationality based on health maintenance and preservation. In reality, there are many other 'rationalities' that influence young people's lives and actions.

Second, the major outcome variables in such approaches are normally the stated intentions of the individual towards a particular behaviour (for example, condom use) and relatively little consideration is given to the relationship between intentions and actions.

Third, the models generally assume a high level of volition amongst young people. This tends to overlook the importance of (a) power dynamics within specific relationships and interactions, (b) structural features that deny (or at least place barriers in the way of) possibilities for action, and (c) the many others who have a strong vested interest in what young people do and do not do – these include parents, teachers, church officials, friends, partners, and others.

Fourth, the analytic demands of such models require a particular form of data-collection in the form of self-completion seven-point rating scales. Their use assumes that all the participants understand the terms in the same way, over-simplifies the range of answers by enforcing circles or crosses as

An example of a study using the Theory of Reasoned Action (TRA)

In 1993, a group of Australian researchers put together an edited collection that explored the application of the Theory of Reasoned Action to HIV prevention behaviour. One of the initial authors of the TRA wrote in the Introduction that '... people turn out to be very good predictors of their own behaviour ... people who intend to perform a given behaviour typically do perform that behaviour.', '... the relative weights of the [attitudinal and normative] components [in predicting intentions] will vary as a function of both the behaviour under consideration and the population being studied' (Fishbein, 1993: xix–xxiii). The theory is represented in figure 3.1.

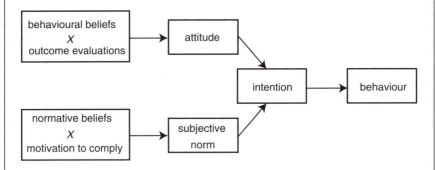

Figure 3.1 The theory of reasoned action

An example of the TRA in application is provided in the volume by Ross and McLaws (1993). In attempting to account for intentions to use condoms amongst 173 men who have sex with men, they used five measures of belief (for example, *condoms are unerotic, condoms interrupt sex, condoms will protect me from infection from the AIDS virus*); each was assessed on a five-point scale and then the score was multiplied by the scores from further five-point scales asking the extent to which respondents were certain or uncertain of their views. The sum of these products formed the attitude measure.

Subjective norms were assessed through scales asking what they thought important others (steady sexual partners, casual sexual partners, close gay friends, people in the community and family) thought about using condoms; these scale scores were again multiplied by the scores regarding the extent to which respondents reported taking notice of these important others. The sum of these products formed the measure of subjective norms.

Using suitable modelling techniques, the authors found that around one-fifth of the variance in stated intentions were accounted for by these measures, with subjective norms being more important than attitudes. A further one-fifth of the variance was accounted for by reported condom use during the two months prior to the study.

responses (for example, there is no place for an 'it all depends' response) and makes invisible other possible dimensions that may be important but that do not fit the particular theoretical model being used. Finally, even where statistical relationships are found between components of the models, these are often quite modest, do not normally permit substantively significant causal relations to be identified nor understanding as to how such attitudes and/or knowledge were derived or can be changed, thereby having little programmatic use.

In recent years, there has been a shift amongst some social scientists and programme developers away from attempting to understand risk and risk behaviour as being solely, or even primarily, determined by individual level attributes towards a greater recognition of the importance of the idea of 'vulnerability'; in other words, the environmental and social contexts that act as levers for, or barriers to, the adoption of healthier lifestyles (Shaw and Aggleton, 2002; Aggleton, 2004).

It would be simple to say that the term 'context' could be used to capture everything that affects young people over and above their individual personal and cognitive attributes. Thus, for example, we could accept that individual attributes are important (albeit challenging to measure accurately) and that wider contexts interact with these to produce an outcome; indeed, many writers adopt just this view. On the other hand, some researchers and programme managers adopt a more structurally deterministic view, and suggest that individual attributes are of marginal significance in understanding the complexities of behaviour (especially in the poorest countries of the world, and among multiply deprived vulnerable groups of young people where the exercise of choice is severely constrained), and that social and physical structures are all-important. The relation between individual actors and the environment in which they live has been hotly debated within social sciences for many years now, and will undoubtedly be so for many years to come. In a nutshell, the key issue is the extent to which we regard young people (and indeed all of us) as being primarily 'agents' or individuals largely constrained and directed by their circumstances.

As ever, such simple dichotomies do not assist us much in understanding how to progress in order to improve the health and welfare of young people. Certainly, emphasising a contextual approach provides a strong warning against the 'injection' model of health improvement, whereby it is felt that if only we could inject the 'right' level of knowledge and the 'right' type of attitudes and skills into individual young people, then all would be well. Whilst these may well be essential, they are by no means sufficient.

Of course, the two levels – the individual and the structural - overlap to a very large extent, so much so that it is almost impossible to assess them separately. To take one example; there has been increasing interest in recent years in the concept of 'discourses' as a means to understand social action. Put simply, 'discourses' are sets of taken-for-granted 'logics' – assumptions that people hold and that guide their actions in particular areas. In some cases, it is felt that there is a range from which we can pick and choose depending on the situation. In other respects, there is a sense in which we are embedded within particular discursive frameworks and cannot stand 'outside' (or escape from) them (see, for example, Parker, 1992; Yardley, 1997).

The relevance of this approach to the focus of this chapter is as follows. The social contexts will to a large extent determine the views and attitudes (the discursive frameworks) of young people and key adults (parents, service providers, teachers, and so on). In other words, the contexts become internalised and any attempt to separate the social from the individual becomes problematic. Sexual identities and practices themselves are socially determined to a large extent, and Gagnon and Simon (1974) drew attention some years ago to the importance of sexual scripts as guides to action. The extent to which different stakeholders can influence discursive frameworks is affected by the power relations that pertain; in general, young people have little relative power.

As an illustration of this approach, Schifter and Madrigal (2000) identified various sexual discourses existing in Costa Rican society in the late 1990s; these include the formal – emanating from scientific rationality, religion and the state – and the informal – rooted in local feminism or romantic love. They illustrate how these are normative, coercive, how they complement and contradict, how they overlap and change, and how they are not politically neutral and can engender resistance. They argue that the power of the state and its close links with religious ideologies ensure that the formal discourses dominate, but bear little relation to the informal level more frequently observed amongst young people. Programmatic efforts – be they in health or education settings, within families, or wherever – stand little chance of success if the various actors are basically speaking different languages. In other societies, one might expect somewhat different discourses to be identified through similar research.

Having said this, we still need to understand what is meant by the term 'context'. As mentioned above, this can be defined in negative terms – that is, what is not 'inside' the individual (even if we accept that what is inside individual heads is contextually determined). In some senses, this definition does capture the way in which the term has been used in the literature; some authors have used a vague notion of 'context' to 'sweep up' anything that is left over after individual factors have been accounted for. Thus, for example, a failure of a particular model to account for much variance in a study can be explained away by reference to 'other' (ill-defined environmental or contextual) factors; in this genre, the basic assumptions of the models themselves are rarely scrutinised.

Others, however, have adopted a more positive definition, recognising the great importance of contextual influences on individual and group action. The range covered is indeed extensive, and a number of different ways of categorising the many different – but overlapping – factors have been developed. At a simple level, one can classify these factors into distal and proximal – the former relate to those that have accumulated within a society or culture over time; examples would be societal norms regarding pre-marital sexual activity, or assumed patterns of dominance and submission within sexual contacts. Proximal contexts refer to the interpersonal situation, in which – at any moment during an interaction – there are factors that will affect outcomes. Examples include the manifestation of gendered power dynamics, or the need for secrecy and possibly hurriedness, both issues that probably affect young people's sexual encounters to a greater extent than those of older people in regular ongoing relationships.

Chalmers et al. (2006) suggest using five elements of contexts that should be considered when exploring young people's sexual health and the factors that may affect it. These are the political context (the legal and policy issues of relevance to the health and education of young people, as well as to legislative issues relating to abuse, rape, stigma and discrimination, and others), the socio-economic context (covering demographic situations and patterns, employment and unemployment issues, educational opportunities, access to services and provisions, and so on), the community context (including the religious, cultural and traditional influences on young people, norms, and so on), the interpersonal context (in which young people live their lives and negotiate their relationships with partners, parents, teachers, and others) and the programmatic context (covering the extent to which, and the style in which, responses to young people's needs occur).

In producing such a classification, the complexity of the relationships between categories must not be under-estimated. The influences of (and on) many of these factors are multi-directional; for example, community norms that proscribe premarital sexual activity may be reflected in the attitudes and behaviour of health service staff so, whereas a dedicated young person's service may be established, the actual experience of accessing it may not be pleasant or welcoming. Similarly, laws and policies do not arise in vacuums; there must be some degree of public and community support for their introduction (see Chapter 12 in this volume), and laws (and codes of conduct) are only as effective as the willingness of people to report breaches and of those charged with implementation to take appropriate action (for example, in the event of rape, or of the sexual harassment of students by lecturers in return for better grades; see, for example, Shumba and Masiki Matina, 2002).

Why understanding and monitoring contexts is so important

High-quality research needs to continue to explore – and improve our understanding of – the complex issues involved in the determination of risk and vulnerability-related behaviours and the ways in which the many different aspects inter-relate. However, the urgency of the situation of HIV and AIDS across the world necessitates action based on best practice consensus even if hard data are sometimes lacking. In such cases, arguments may need to be based on human rights perspectives; in general, these are highly consistent with the emerging research data.

As mentioned earlier, and despite the conceptual difficulties of 'separating' individuals from the contexts in which they live, it is crucial to develop means by which contexts and changes can be monitored, and their impacts assessed. There are a number of reasons why this is important. Even for those who prefer to work with individual level data – such as can be derived from knowledge, attitudes, behaviour and practices (KAPB) surveys – or those who are limited to such data – such as behavioural surveillance surveys – a great deal still needs to be explained. For example, attitudes and subjective norms (as used in the Theory of Reasoned Action, for example) or perceived behavioural control (as used in the Theory of Planned Behaviour) or frequency of condom use, do not arise in a vacuum; they derive from somewhere. This 'somewhere' may be located in family contexts, school-based sex education, media coverage of sexuality, and so on. More sophisticated models demand even more explanation.

After a comprehensive review of the literature, coupled with detailed analysis of qualitative material gained from individual interviews in the UK and the Netherlands, a framework was developed to try to capture the many and varied influences that appear to affect sexual outcomes (Vanwesenbeeck et al., 1999). The core of the process was the actual (or potential) sexual interaction, and some of the distal (background and intermediate) and proximal variables that have been found to affect this are incorporated into the framework. These 'variables' and the relationships between them are complex, and the framework serves to illustrate a number of levels at which distal and proximal contexts influence outcomes. In turn, each of the 'explanatory' variables is itself subject to, and determined by, a complex set of factors. Two parallel pathways in the framework reflect the fact that the two people involved each arrive at the interaction with their own particular sets of histories, skills, knowledge, attitudes, and so on, which have been affected by their backgrounds (or the contexts in which they have developed).

There is a need to identify barriers to improved sexual and reproductive health. Much of the past emphasis has been on young people as risk takers (encouraged by the extensive use of KAPB instruments). Comparatively less emphasis has been directed towards those who determine policies that actively or passively discourage the very conditions under which improved sexual health can be achieved. From this perspective, one sometimes has to ask 'just who are the risk-takers?' Through a greater awareness of the ways in which different contexts encourage or discourage, or enable or deny, particular discourses and activities, then we can identify where the barriers exist and continue the attempts to address them.

Drawing attention to contexts helps to shift the emphasis away from an 'individual deficit' model of young people and to encourage others to accept that there are many levels of responsibility in the efforts to improve sexual health in general, and to combat HIV and AIDS in particular. Indeed, there are few, if any, sectors of societies that do not, directly or indirectly, have important implications for the health of young people. Encouraging a collective responsibility for a nation's ill-health must be an important target.

Articles within the various relevant UN Conventions (for example, the Convention on the Rights of the Child [UN, 1989]), declarations (for example, against violence to women [UN, 1993] and the International Conference on Population and Development (ICPD) and ICPD+5 agreements [UN, 1994, 1999]) and within UN system agencies' strategic frameworks and technical working documents (for example, UNAIDS, 2002) refer to the need to establish appropriate contexts in the fields of health, education, employment, the legal system, anti-discrimination, and others. In some cases, these contexts will be developed through laws, in others through policies, and in yet others through trying to change social norms through education in different settings. Whichever apply, the success or otherwise with which countries or regions are achieving these aims (and/or fulfilling their obligations) needs to be monitored closely.

Some problems in knowing 'what works'

There is an appealing simplicity about assessing 'what works' in terms of interventions to improve sexual health. 'Measurement' of some attribute – such as knowledge, attitudes, intentions to use condoms, recent condom use, age at first intercourse, numbers of partners, and so on – can be performed before the intervention and again afterwards, enabling the impact to be assessed. Regrettably, life (and programmatic implementation) is not so simple.

There have been various attempts to isolate the impact of one or other form of intervention (using randomised control trials) but these are fraught with methodological and theoretical difficulties, quite apart from being very expensive to conduct. For example, a school-based sex education programme may be designed in an effort to alter the ways in which young people begin to engage on their sexual lives. Such a programme might cover knowledge, values, gender norms, communication and negotiation skills through role-plays, etc. An evaluation of the impact of such a programme might show no impact, and so a conclusion might erroneously be reached (and probably would be by some family-oriented campaigners) that school sex education is ineffective, when in fact it may have been the context surrounding the intervention that reduced its potential impact.

Young people live in a variety of contexts; they live within families of one kind or another, may live with natural parents or surrogate parents, the 'atmosphere' within the home may be open or closed with regard to sexuality, they may be linked with religious organisations, they will have peer groups outside of school, and so on. In other words, they inhabit and are affected by a wide range of contexts, some of which may provide contradictory levels of support for acting in certain ways. If the needs for survival, or material goods, or reputations, or affection, and so on are strong then these contexts may well outweigh any others that have been encouraged. In this sense, the school-based programme outlined above is just one of a range of – possibly contradictory – contexts.

A further issue to bear in mind when considering possible links between independent variables and dependent variables is that what has an impact in one country and/or society (and/or sector) may not do so in another. There are many reasons for this, including those mentioned above. Further, it is possible that the same contexts may have different impacts depending on the stage of the epidemic, as well as on other aspects of young people's lives. Thus, a search for the magic contextual formula that may be applied across all settings is probably doomed to fail.

As an alternative to the search for the 'magic intervention', some authors have instead considered constellations of factors and argued that these can be shown to have an impact on outcomes. What they cannot say with any certainty is what precisely has an effect. Three examples are provided here, each using material from relatively well-developed countries.

A comprehensive study sponsored by the Alan Guttmacher Institute considered a range of industrialised countries (Jones *et al.*, 1985). They developed a range of indices of sexual 'openness' (including condom availability, condom advertising, contraceptive services for unmarried young people, sex education in schools, and so on) and correlated these with a range of outcome indicators, the main one being teenage conception rates. They found that the higher the cumulative score of 'openness', the lower the rate of teenage conceptions.

A more recent follow-up to this study using just five countries (the USA, Great Britain, Sweden, France and Canada) produced generally similar results (Singh *et al.*, 2001). As well as pointing out how important social and economic disadvantage are in affecting teenage conceptions rates, the authors point out that, at all socioeconomic levels,

> ... societal acceptance of sexual activity among young people, combined with comprehensive and balanced information about sexuality ... are hallmarks of countries with low levels of adolescent pregnancy, childbearing and STDs ... Easy access to contraceptives and other reproductive health services in Sweden, France, Canada and Great Britain contributes to better contraception use and therefore lower teenage pregnancy rates than in the US. Easy access means that adolescents know where to obtain information and services, can reach a

provider easily, are assured of receiving confidential, non-judgmental care, and can obtain services and contraceptive supplies at little or no cost

(Singh *et al.*, 2001: 1)

An analysis of a much larger range of countries drawn from four continents has been carried out by UNICEF and published in their Report Card series. Detailed analyses of birth data from 28 OECD countries are presented and recent trends are discussed. The report concludes that those countries that have successfully reduced rates are characterised by both motivation and means. 'Motivation' here refers to the extent to which young people feel a stake in the future, a sense of hope and an expectation of inclusion. The 'means'

> ... involve not only the degree of availability of contraception, but also the kind of sex education which enables young people to make informed and mutually-respectful choices, including the choice to delay having sex or to insist on safe contraception.
>
> (UNICEF, 2001: 25)

Of course, one needs to be very careful extrapolating from these analyses of 'richer' countries to other settings in 'poorer' countries. Nevertheless, the results do indicate that somewhat greater understanding can be achieved through considering these comprehensive contexts than through consideration of isolated interventions.

What is clear, however, is that the general pattern revealed across these countries in terms of better sexual health is highly consistent both with the direction of Human Rights Conventions, as well as the relatively little comparable data that exist from poorer countries. For example, the relative success of countries such as Brazil, Uganda and Zambia in reducing the rates of new HIV infections among young people is generally acknowledged as being due to a greater level of public acceptance of there being a problem to be faced, supported by improved services and targeted prevention campaigns (UNAIDS, 2000a; Singh *et al.*, 2003). There is now widespread acceptance in the field as to the general direction in which progress is required (except amongst some religious and political organisations) which should assist in identifying the sorts of contextual factors that need to be addressed.

Some problems of measurement and methods

There may be general agreement on the required direction, but there are some problems when we get down to specifics. Accurate data on HIV prevalence are hard to obtain, STI rates are affected by patterns of clinic attendance and diagnosis (which in turn are affected by the availability and accessibility of services, staff attitudes, whether symptoms are present or not, individual motivations towards health care, and so on), the numbers of unintended conceptions may be concealed through unregistered abortions, infanticide, and so on. Furthermore, many countries – when they do record data – do not disaggregate these into age groups.

So, there are serious problems in assessing the outcomes that may arise within particular contexts. Equally, however, there are problems in assessing contexts. Certainly, the numbers of young people oriented clinics can be counted, but this will say little about the quality of the service provided. Similarly, the existence of a national sex and relationships education curriculum can be identified, but this will say little about the extent to which the course materials are gathering dust on head teachers' shelves, and/or whether individual teachers adumbrate the material with particular moralistic slants.

More general areas pose similar problems. For example, if societal 'openness' regarding sexual issues in general, or HIV in particular, is regarded as an important contextual attribute (as indicated in the studies mentioned above), how exactly is this to be assessed? Asking a number of key informants may produce a range of contrasting responses which may well be affected by their experiences elsewhere, their moral standpoints, their discursive frameworks, and so on. Analysing media campaigns can be done by recording the numbers of advertising slots (or soap opera hours) devoted to HIV-relevant issues but may tell us little about who has access to the material, within what social circumstances they view them, how well they understand the messages, how relevant they feel them to be to themselves personally, and a range of other issues.

In other words, the monitoring of some apparently obvious areas for inclusion is not as simple as it may at first appear. Adults may (and often do) feel that they have created an appropriate context for young people to develop and foster, but the young people's views may not be compatible with those of the adults involved. Furthermore, different adults may have differing intentions – those of parents may well differ from those of teachers, religious leaders, doctors, and others. This raises questions as to the usefulness of the normal criteria of reliability and validity of these kinds of measures; if contexts are assessed in different ways by different people, then whose interpretation is to be afforded priority? One of the major epistemological contributions of the discursive approach advocated here has been to draw into serious question the notion of a 'truth' that needs to be discovered, and against which our measuring instruments need to be validated. Of course, self-reported behaviour can (in theory at least) be validated against biological markers of infection, but life is not so straightforward when considering the rather more nebulous concept of contextual influences.

This leads on to the question of methods. Clearly, a range of methods is available to assess key elements of, and change in, contexts depending on the specific indices to be selected. But the costs and feasibility of specific modes of enquiry need to be considered; so, for example, regular monitoring of the circumstances of first ever intercourse (in terms of reasons, coercion, transactional aspects, subsequent regret, and so on) requires large and well chosen samples to ensure that adequate comparisons can be made both between (and within) countries and across time. Comparisons across countries (and between different linguistic groups within countries) are notoriously difficult through questionnaires, both in terms of language and comprehension, but also in terms of anchoring the end-points of the scales used; for example, what is regarded as being 'extreme' pressure in one country may be regarded as being rather mild within another.

Assessing policy aspects may need to rely on broadly qualitative approaches through, for example, interviewing or conducting focus group discussions with key informants at various levels in the process (ministers, civil servants, local council officers, local staff, and so on). Again, problems of comparability and repeatability arise; these will be exacerbated by sampling problems and also by the partial perceptions of the different people sampled. For example, the Department for International Development (DfID) supported *Safe Passages to Adulthood* programme developed an approach to Dynamic Contextual Analyses (Chalmers *et al.*, 2001, revised in Chalmers *et al.*, 2006) and carried out pilot studies in six countries; in some countries, researchers were assured by fairly senior key informants that good policies were in place in one or another area. However, when data were collected from those working nearer the ground, a rather different picture emerged (summary reports are available on the SPA website, www.safepassages.sofon.ac.uk). The different actors in the process of policy formulation and implementation have different experiences and different vested interests. Furthermore, their own personal views on young people's sexual activity may colour the responses received.

Some suggested ways forward

The potential problems in collecting suitable data for the purpose of monitoring contextual influences should not act as deterrents from the task. It is, however, important to ensure that any data collected are meaningful and relevant to the task in hand, and not just collected for the sake of it. Some guides have been produced in recent years to assist this task (for example, UNAIDS, 2000b; Webb and Elliott, 2000; Makinwa and O'Grady, 2001; Hawkins and Price, nd; Boyce *et al.*, 2004; Malcolm and Aggleton, 2004).

Kirby (2001), writing in the context of programmes designed to reduce teen pregnancy rates in the USA, makes the useful distinction between those that focus on sexual antecedents and those that focus on non-sexual antecedents. Whilst some may wish to argue with his use of the term 'antecedent' (with its implication of simple cause and effect mechanisms), the distinction is relevant to the present discussion.

There is much evidence that, in most if not all countries, those most vulnerable to poorer sexual health are those who are the most excluded from education and employment – addressing such factors would fall under what Kirby calls 'non-sexual antecedents'. Thus, general contexts in terms of the proportions of young men and women who receive basic and secondary education, who are in employment, who live below the poverty line and so on, should be routinely recorded. Such data are, for the most part, available from existing UN sources (for example, UNFPA, 2003). However, the impact of poverty and other reasons for exclusion are mediated through various processes, so a more specific emphasis on contexts most directly related to sexual health is justified.

In considering the issues involved in the creation and maintenance of appropriate contexts, it is useful to introduce a distinction between three levels at which impacts might be expected. For the sake of simplicity, these have been termed macro, intermediate and micro. Macro is used to refer to national or regional policies; the key question here is whether there are policies in place that are consistent with what is known about the development of contexts that are conducive to improving the task of HIV prevention. Intermediate is concerned with the steps that are needed in terms of implementing the policy into practice; for example, a national policy regarding improved sex and relationships education in schools will require that teachers are trained sufficiently well to deliver it and that course materials are available and accessible. Finally, micro refers to the level of face-to-face interactions in the range of settings in which young people live; to continue the example above, whether the training of teachers translates into actual improved practice in the classroom and, in turn, whether and how this improved practice translates into safer sexual activity amongst the students. Note though, that national policies do not necessarily need to be in place in a particular area for the other levels to be relevant and applicable; local initiatives can be (and of course have been) taken by enlightened individuals and/or organisations without waiting for national guidelines and leadership.

As well as this (to some extent) artificial means of dividing the world into levels, there is a further set of distinctions to be made. We can consider the challenges in terms of formal structures (education and health systems, for example) and informal structures (leisure activities, localised social worlds, and so on), and we can also think in terms of cross-cutting issues (gender relations, discrimination and stigma, rights, consistency in discourses encountered, and so on). Relying on just the former of these dimensions runs the risk of splitting up the world up in this way, diverts attention away from the need for 'joined-up' thinking, and gives priority to aspects of organisational structures and processes rather than to young people's perspectives. On the other hand, the cross-cutting issues are far harder to measure and a sole reliance on these may be regarded by some as being too vague or 'slippery' to be useful. The challenge lies in developing ways of understanding and developing indices that pay due recognition to the maximum number of relevant aspects.

Applying these dimensions, and in order to try to capture the complexity in a reasonably understandable way, a conceptual cube can be developed. This is shown (for ease of representation) as two grids, as in Tables 3.1 and 3.2. Table 3.1 lists some of the formal and informal contexts against the levels at which they operate and includes, within each cell, some of the issues that need to be addressed. The second grid (Table 3.2) introduces the cross-cutting issues. The third face of the cube represents the three levels of potential influence.

The text in the cells merely provides examples of the sorts of issues that can and should be considered under each heading and within the various contexts. Each of these (and many others not provided here as examples) can be fleshed out to develop research and monitoring agendas.

The task of assessing this wide range of contexts and their possible impact is highly challenging. A range of approaches needs to be used as appropriate for the task in hand, including analysis of survey data (although additional questions to those commonly used may be required), interviews with key informants including, of course, young people, collection and analysis of relevant statistics, desk analysis of policy and strategy documents, media outlets, and so on. Documents and texts can be analysed at the simple levels of content and themes, through to full discourse analysis (Potter and Wetherell, 1987; Parker, 1992).

Contained within the examples provided in the figures is a distinction between what might be called the 'outsiders' perspective and that of the 'insiders'. In this case, the 'insiders' will be young people in general, or a particular sub-set, such as women, those who are same-sex attracted, drug users, and so on. The 'outsiders' will be all those others who have a role in setting and determining the contexts in which the insiders live their lives. Examples of the sorts of issues that might be investigated in relation to policy development are:

From the outsiders' perspective – what are the formal policy and legal positions (the extent of policies and laws governing HIV/AIDS and/or sex and relationship education, accessible and available health service provision for young people, anti-discrimination (gender and HIV status), and so on)? Do the policies include all young people (those not attending school and particularly vulnerable young people, for example)? Do the policies reflect human rights issues (is there specific mention of young people's rights)? Is there high-level public support for these policies (has the national president or some other suitable high status person made a public declaration of support for improving young people's sexual health and/or increased efforts to

Table 3.1 A conceptual framework for assessing contexts (part one)

	Education	Health	Workplace	Family or substitute	Religions	Media
Macro-level	are there national policies in place regarding sex education and HIV education? are there policies for non-attenders?	is there a planned development of young people's sexual health services? are there confidentiality policies? policies for outreach?	are there anti-discrimination policies in place? is there a policy for treatment and care?	is there national support for parental involvement in sex-and-relationships education and support?	international or national policies on prevention? international or national policies on treatment and care? accuracy of information provided?	accessibility of different media?
Intermediate level	training for teachers? pre-service? in-service? printed curricula? age at delivery? style of delivery? outreach work?	training for work with young people? accessibility? provision of free or affordable contraception? targeted work for marginalised groups? quality of record-keeping?	is HIV training provided for the workforce? are policies enforced?	training and support for parents and carers in sexual health matters?	implementation of policies?	issues dealt with sensibly and without sensationalism? images of men and women, people living with HIV, diversity, etc.?
Micro-level	implementation? regular evaluation by young people?	usage of services by young people? evaluation by young people?	feelings of safety and acceptance	extent of open and honest communication on sexual issues?		influence on social norms within relevant groups? opportunity to seek advice and support?

Table 3.2 A conceptual framework for assessing contexts (part two)

	Stigma and discrimination	Socio-economic issues	Gender issues	Consistency of approach
Macro-level	are there policies/laws in place to prevent discrimination against people living with or affected by HIV? ditto for sexual orientation	do policies and laws take into account all sectors of society?	are there national policies/laws concerning equal rights? are there national policies/laws on sexual abuse and coercion?	do laws and policies from different departments conflict?
Intermediate level	training for relevant staff to ensure these policies are practised? attempts at tackling prejudice and myths about HIV?	are special efforts made to reach poorer and/or marginalised and/or more vulnerable groups?	training for all relevant staff on projects working with young women and men? are breaches suitably dealt with?	are different structures integrated (for example, health services on or near to school sites)?
Micro-level	absence of stigma and discrimination feelings of safety	connection to community	mutuality and respect in relationships fewer coercive sexual relationships	ready access at convenient times and locations

combat HIV)? What are/were the processes through which policies are/were developed and monitored (who was involved, were/are young people consulted)? This list is not exhaustive and there are other key questions to be asked as well.

From the insider's perspective, key questions to be asked include: do all young people feel that they have a supportive environment in relation to their sexual health and relationship concerns, or do certain groups feel excluded from educational opportunities and/or health service provision? Are contraceptive supplies and advice readily available and affordable (how far to the nearest supplier, can young people afford to buy them)? Do young people feel that they can have their questions answered honestly and openly (by parents, health staff, teachers, helplines, Internet access, and/or others)? Do young people who are attracted to others of the same sex feel that they are stigmatised? Do young women feel that they are pressured into sexual activity against their wishes (what reasons are given by young people for engaging in early sex, do they report regret after the event)? Do young men feel pressured into sexual activity against their wishes (ditto as above)? Do young people whose lives are directly affected by HIV/AIDS feel stigmatised or supported (including people living with HIV/AIDS, orphans, carers, and so on)?

Assessment of contexts (in this example, the existence of appropriate policies) that rely solely on the outsider's perspective will be severely lacking if they are not 'triangulated' to ensure that the intended effect is acknowledged by the target groups involved. When points of commonality emerge, then it is clear that the policies are relatively well-tuned to the needs of the young people involved. However, where differences are found, action of some form needs to be taken. It may be, for example, that those charged with setting policies are, for one or more reasons, simply not in tune with the genuine needs of young people; perhaps they do not take monitoring and evaluation seriously enough, possibly they have developed or maintained policies that are designed to serve purposes other than supporting young people (for example, to win votes in a forthcoming election), maybe they are driven by a religious or cultural agenda that essentially disregards the realities of being a young person in an increasingly sexualised society, and so on.

Conceptualising and assessing contexts is no easy task, and the scale of the challenge is immense. But this should not deter efforts to enquire into aspects of the complex and enigmatic world in which young people (and we all) live, in which they are exposed to all manner of threats, and in which they struggle to make sense of often conflicting and disingenuous messages. To continue to focus the bulk of research attention on their supposed individual deficits is to do them no favours at all.

References

Aggleton, P. (2004) Sexuality, HIV prevention, vulnerability and risk, *Journal of Psychology and Human Sexuality*, 16(1), 1–11.

Ajzen, I. and Madden, T.J. (1986) Prediction of goal-directed behaviour: Attitudes, intentions and perceived behavioural control, *Journal of Experimental Social Psychology*, 22, 453–74.

Boyce, P., Aggleton, P. and Malcolm, A. (2004) *Rapid Assessment and Response: Adaptation guide on HIV and men who have sex with men*, Geneva: World Health Organisation (available at <www.who.int/entity/hiv/pub/prev_care/en/msmrar.pdf>).

Chalmers, H., Stone, N. and Ingham, R. (2001) *Dynamic Contextual Analysis of Young People's Sexual Health*, Centre for Sexual Health Research, University of Southampton: Safe Passages to Adulthood programme.

Chalmers, H., Aggleton, P., Ingham, R. and Stone, N. (2006) *Dynamic Contextual Analysis of Young People's Sexual Health* (2nd edition), Centre for Sexual Health Research, University of Southampton: Safe Passages to Adulthood programme.

Cleland, J. and Ferry, B. (eds) (1995) *Sexual Behaviour and AIDS in the Developing World*, London: Taylor and Francis.

Fishbein, M. (1993) Introduction, in D. Terry, C. Gallois and M. McCamish (eds) *The Theory of Reasoned Action: Its application to AIDS-preventive behaviour*, Oxford: Pergamon Press, xv–xxv.

Fishbein, M. and Ajzen, I. (1975) *Belief, Attitude, Intention and Behavior: An introduction to theory and method*, Reading MA: Addison-Wesley.

Gagnon, J. and Simon, W. (1974) *Sexual Conduct: The social sources of human sexuality*, London: Hutchinson.

Hawkins, K. and Price, N. (nd) *The Social Context of Sexual and Reproductive Health: A framework for social analysis and monitoring*, University of Swansea: Centre for Development Studies.

Ingham, R. (1994) Some speculations on the concept of rationality, in Albrecht, G. (ed.) *Advances in Medical Sociology, Vol. IV: A reconsideration of models of health behaviour change*, Greenwich: CN, JAI Press, 89–111.

Ingham, R., Woodcock, A. and Stenner, K. (1992) The limitations of rational decision making models as applied to young people's sexual behaviour, in Aggleton, P., Davies, P. and Hart, G. (eds) *AIDS: Rights, risk and reason*, London: Falmer Press, 163–73.

Ingham, R. and van Zessen, G. (1997) Towards an alternative model of sexual behaviour; from individual properties to interactional processes, in Van Campenhoudt, L., Cohen, M., Guizzardi, G. and Hausser, D. (eds) *Sexual Interactions and HIV Risk: New conceptual perspectives in European research*, London: Taylor and Francis, 83–99.

Jones, E., Forrest, J., Goldman, N., Henshaw, S., Lincoln, R., Rossoff, J., Westhoff, C. and Wolf, D. (1985) Teenage pregnancy in developed countries: Determinants and policy implications, *Family Planning Perspectives*, 17 (2), 53–63.

Kippax, S. and Crawford, J. (1993) Flaws in the theory of reasoned action, in D. Terry, C. Gallois and M. McCamish (eds) *The Theory of Reasoned Action: Its application to AIDS-preventive behaviour*, Oxford: Pergamon Press, 253–69.

Kirby, D. (2001) *Emerging Answers: Research findings on programs to reduce teen pregnancy,* Washington DC: National Campaign to Reduce Teen Pregnancy.

Malcolm, A. and Aggleton, P. (2004) *Rapid Assessment and Response: Adaptation guide for work with especially vulnerable young people,* Geneva: World Health Organisation (available at www.who.int/hiv/pub/prev_care/guide/en/print.html).

Makinwa, B. and O'Grady, M. (eds) (2001) *Best Practices in HIV/AIDS Prevention Collection,* Arlington VA/Geneva: FHI/UNAIDS.

Norman, P. and Conner, M. (1995) *Predicting Health Behaviour,* Buckingham, UK: Open University Press.

Parker, I. (1992) *Discourse Dynamics: Critical analysis for social and individual psychology,* London: Routledge.

Potter, J. and Wetherell, M. (1987) *Discourse and Social Psychology: Beyond attitudes and behaviour,* London: Sage.

Rosenstock, I.M., Strecher, V.J. and Becker, M.H. (1988) Social learning theory and the health belief model, *Health Education Quarterly,* 15, 175–83.

Ross, M.W. and McLaws, M-L. (1993) Attitudes towards condoms and the theory of reasoned action, in D. Terry, C. Gallois and M. McCamish (eds) *The Theory of Reasoned Action: Its application to AIDS-preventive behaviour,* Oxford: Pergamon Press, 81–92.

Schifter, J. and Madrigal, J. (2000) *The Sexual Construction of Latino Youth: Implications for the spread of AIDS,* New York: The Haworth Press, Inc.

Shaw, C. and Aggleton, P. (2002) *Preventing HIV/AIDS and Promoting Sexual Health among Especially Vulnerable Young People,* Southampton/Geneva: Safe Passages to Adulthood/WHO.

Sheeran, P., Abraham, C. and Orbell, S. (1999) Psychosocial correlates of heterosexual condom use: A meta-analysis, *Psychological Bulletin,* 125, 1, 90–132.

Shumba, A. and Masiki Matina, A.E. (2002) Sexual harassment of college students by lecturers in Zimbabwe, *Sex Education,* 2, 1, 45–60.

Singh, S., Darroch, J.E. and Frost, J.J. (2001) Socioeconomic disadvantage and adolescent women's sexual and reproductive health: The case of five developed countries. *Family Planning Perspectives,* 33(6) 251–8 and 289.

Singh, S., Darroch, J. and Bankole, A. (2003) *A, B and C in Uganda: The roles of abstinence, monogamy and condom use in HIV decline,* Occasional Report No. 9, December 2003. New York: Alan Guttmacher Institute.

UN (1994) *Population and Development, Vol. 1: Programme of action adopted at the International Conference on Population and Development* (ICPD), Cairo, 5–13 September. New York: Department of Economic and Social Information and Policy Analysis, United Nations.

UN (1999) *Key Actions of the Further Implementation of the Programme of Action of the International Conference on Population and Development,* (A/S-21/5/Add.1) (ICPD+5). New York: United Nations.

UN (1989) *UN Convention on the Rights of the Child,* Geneva: UN High Commission for Human Rights.

UN (1993) *Declaration on the Elimination of Violence against Women,* Geneva: UN High Commission for Human Rights.

UNAIDS (1999) *Summary Booklet of Best Practice, Issue 1,* Geneva: UNAIDS (UNAIDS/99.28E).

UNAIDS (2000a) *Report on the Global HIV/AIDS Epidemic,* Geneva: UNAIDS.

UNAIDS (2000b) *National AIDS Programmes: A guide to monitoring and evaluation*, Geneva: UNAIDS (UNAIDS/00.17E).

UNAIDS (2002) *HIV/AIDS and Education: A strategic approach*, draft report, Geneva: UNAIDS Inter Agency Task Team on Education.

UNFPA (2003) *State of the World's Population: Investing in adolescent's needs and rights*, New York: UNFPA.

UNICEF (2001) *A League Table of Teenage Births in Rich Nations*, Innocenti Report Card No. 3. Florence: UNICEF Innocenti Research Centre.

Vanwesenbeeck, I., van Zessen, G., Ingham, R., Jaramazovic, E. and Stevens, D., (1999) Factors and processes in heterosexual competence and risk: An integrated review of the evidence, *Psychology and Health*, 14 (1), 25–50.

Webb, D. and Elliott, L. (2000) *Learning to Live: Monitoring and evaluating HIV/AIDS programmes for young people*, London: Save the Children UK.

Yardley, L. (ed.) (1997) *Material Discourses of Health and Illness*, London: Routledge.

Chapter 4

Gender, sexual behaviour and vulnerability among young people

Christine Ricardo, Gary Barker,
Julie Pulerwitz and Valéria Rocha

Introduction

Gender – defined here as the socially constructed roles, identities and attributes of men and women – is recognised as a key issue for understanding the sexual behaviour and vulnerabilities of young people (Mensch *et al.*, 1998; WHO, 2000; UNFPA, 2005). Furthermore, it is increasingly acknowledged that gender needs to be taken into account when developing programmes in the area of sexual health (Boender *et al.*, 2004; Schueller *et al.*, 2005). However, gender is a complex concept, and this complexity is seldom taken into account during programme planning and implementation. Indeed, in most initiatives, gender is seen as an external factor, beyond the scope of direct intervention, or is acknowledged as an important cross-cutting issue, but is not addressed explicitly or directly.

In addition, discussions of gender have often focused exclusively on the challenges facing young women, too often ignoring the gender-specific vulnerabilities of men and boys. Although young women are generally more at risk of health and development problems, young men in most places suffer from higher morbidity and mortality rates, and are disproportionately perpetrators and victims of violence, with the exception of sexual violence (WHO, 2000). Furthermore, in the last decade, there has been a growing international consensus regarding the key role that men and boys play in empowering women and girls and achieving gender equality as reflected in a series of milestone meetings and documents, including the 1994 International Conference on Population and Development (UNFPA, 1994) and the 1995 Fourth World Conference on Women (UN, 1995).

In this chapter, we illustrate how gender represents a complex interplay of contextual and individual factors, which create advantages and disadvantages for both young women and young men in terms of sexuality and related health issues. We apply an ecological model to emphasise how gender norms, as they relate to sexual behaviour, are internalised by the individual through an interaction of factors including cognitive processes, relationships with family, peer groups, intimate partners, and access to and quality of available social supports, services, and policies. Based on this discussion, we also highlight examples of how programmes can successfully operationalise strategies that address gender and identify some promising programme directions.

Gender and the construction of sexuality

Gender shapes attitudes and behaviours related to sexuality by the different norms and expectations it imparts on young women and young men. For young women, there continue to be strict socio-cultural norms in many settings regarding their sexuality, particularly relating to virginity before marriage and numbers of sexual partners (Weiss and Gupta, 1998). Puberty may bring marked attention to a young woman's ability to reproduce and, in some cultures, may signal a period of greater social exclusion, more attention to movements outside the home and more protection from boys (Mensch *et al.*, 1998). At the same time, between 10 and 60 per cent of women report having had premarital sex in surveys conducted in poorer countries around the world (Mensch *et al.*, 1998). Underlying these statistics are several contextual factors, including the influence of norms on the accurate reporting of female sexual activity, the extent of non-consensual relations, as well as an increased sexual assertiveness amongst young women in many settings.

Moreover, it is important to consider the role of rigid gender norms in reinforcing violence and impacting upon unsafe sexual behaviour. Often considered the most disturbing form of traditional gender roles and unequal power distribution, violence against women underlies a great part of women's vulnerability to sexual and reproductive health problems, including HIV infection (Heise *et al.*, 1999). Research from around the world has also shown that sexual initiation is involuntary for many girls (Jejeebhoy and Bott, 2003). In a recent population-based survey in the Caribbean, nearly 50 per cent of young women (between the ages of 10 and 18 years) reported that their first sexual experience was 'forced' or 'somewhat forced' (UN Millennium Project, 2005). Furthermore, some research has found that sexual coercion is more common in settings where traditional gender roles of masculinity and dominance are more rigid (Heise, 1998).

Research also suggests that many young women have been socialised to accept male control of sexual decision-making (Jejeebhoy and Bott, 2003). A study in South Africa found that young women identified their ideal relationship as one in which the male made the decisions, including the use of condoms and the timing of sex (Harrison *et al.*, 2001). Among 11- to 15-year-old school-going young people in Jamaica, 69 per cent of boys and 32 per cent of girls agreed with the statement that 'if you really love your [partner], you should have sex with them' and more than half (58 per cent) of boys and 30 per cent of girls said that if a boy 'spends a lot of money on a girl' she should have sex with him (Eggleston and Hardee, 1999).

Although young men's sexual experiences are, in general, more self-determined than those of women, it is important to acknowledge the extent to which gender norms and social pressures influence how they act in intimate relationships. Boys or young men who display their emotions or who show interest in caring or domestic roles might be ridiculed by peers and others in the community as being 'sissies' or not 'real men'; in this way, societal expectation might restrict their ability to see themselves as caring, non-violent and responsible partners (UNFPA, 2000).

For many young men worldwide, sexual experience is frequently associated with initiation into a socially recognised manhood. In much of Africa, for example, there are explicit rites of passage where much attention is given to boys' needs to become sexually active and to prove they have achieved an adult version of manhood. This fosters a perception of sex as performance, specifically a means by which to demonstrate masculine prowess. Sexual experiences may be viewed among peers as displays of sexual competence or accomplishment, rather than acts of intimacy (Marsiglio, 1988; Nzioka, 2001). This pattern of sexual bravado as a means to peer acceptance often continues into manhood (Khan *et al.*, 1998).

Gender affects sexuality not just for heterosexual men and women, but also for same-sex or bi-sexually attracted men and women, and it is clearly linked to homophobia. For boys and young men in much of the world, homophobia is often part of gender socialisation and sexual roles. Often, boys are enjoined to act in certain ways, or risk being stigmatised by being labelled homosexual or gay (Rivers and Aggleton, 1999). For young men who are gay, or who have sex with men, this stigmatisation can lead them to practice their sexuality clandestinely and inhibit them from seeking out sexual health information and services, thus creating situations of extreme vulnerability to STIs and HIV. Furthermore, due to this stigmatisation, health services and regular sexual education programmes might not be welcoming to same-sex or bi-sexually attracted young men and young women or might not be prepared to deal with questions and concerns related to sexual diversity.

The complexities of gender: using an ecological model to discuss gender-specific vulnerabilities

An ecological framework can be used to map the dynamic interrelationships with family, peers, structural factors and wider socio-cultural norms that impact the behaviours, and vulnerability, of both young men and young women (Sallis and Owen, 2002). These interrelationships are commonly portrayed as multiple levels of factors that influence the development, attitudes and behaviours of the individual, who is represented at the centre. It is important to note that there have been various descriptions and applications of ecological models (for example, Bronfenbrenner, 1979; McLeroy *et al.,* 1988). For the purpose of our discussion, we will use an ecological model that highlights how socio-cultural, structural, inter-personal and individual factors are relevant for understanding and addressing gender-specific vulnerabilities.

In the outer level of this ecological model is the macro-environment. This encompasses the larger culture, which, we would argue, permeates throughout all levels of the model and influences interactions between the individual and different contextual factors. Our discussion of the macro-environment here will focus on socio-cultural norms around gender. The next level in the model can be described as a grouping of community and structural factors that includes access to and quality of institutions such as schools, religious centres, health clinics and non-governmental organisations (NGOs). For our discussion of this level, we will highlight how socio-economic opportunities, access to and quality of health services, and policy help shape the gender-specific vulnerabilities of young women and young men in terms of sexuality and health.

In the level closest to the individual, or most direct level of influence, are family and peers. At the centre is the individual young woman and young man, whose development in relation to their gender-specific vulnerabilities is a confluence of dynamic interactions across the multiple levels of the model.

In this discussion, we will start with socio-cultural norms and move inwards toward the individual. However, the interactions of the different levels in the model are dynamic and multi-directional and, just as socio-cultural norms help to shape the attitudes and behaviours of young women and young men, so do these young people, in turn, help to construct socio-cultural norms. As articulated by Diffusion of Innovations (DOI) theory, it is a critical mass, or tipping point, of changes in the attitudes and behaviours of individuals that can catalyse a process of change in societal norms (Rogers, 1995; White *et al.,* 2003).

Socio-cultural norms

Gender is the set of social roles and symbolic meanings accorded to males and females. As a concept, gender helps us understand how social relations are hierarchical and asymmetrical, how they produce unequal power relations, and how they interact with other factors, such as age, religion, sexuality, race and social class. For example, not only do many aspects of the masculine identity frequently constrain young men and make them more vulnerable to certain high-risk situations, there are at times interactions with other variables that might prove even more constraining. For example, young bisexual or homosexual men may be subject to discrimination from male peers, which can have a direct impact on their decision to seek information or support regarding HIV prevention. Similarly, a low-income young woman has a much lower chance of having access to proper medical and neonatal care than a financially well-to-do woman, thus increasing chances of morbidity or death to her and/or her newborn baby.

Numerous researchers have affirmed that gender norms are among the strongest underlying social factors that influence sexual behaviours, including violence against women (Gupta, 2000; Varga, 2003). The internalisation of gender norms happens through a process of socialisation with family, peer groups and communities in a dynamic, bidirectional interaction with the individual. This internalisation often defines how men and women treat each other in relationships and has substantial implications for the nature of sexual relations (Rivers and Aggleton, 1999; Varga, 2003). For example, boys are often raised to meet an ideal of masculinity characterised by being aggressive and competitive, and during 'adolescence' they often gain more autonomy and mobility to fulfil the masculine mandate of being successful providers and protectors. By contrast, ideals of femininity often dictate that women be sexually coy and passive with partners.

We would also like to clarify that although the emphasis of this chapter is the construction of gender norms as a key issue in the sexual behaviour and vulnerabilities of young people, we acknowledge that it is not the only issue that shapes young people's sexual behaviours and vulnerability – race, ethnicity and social class, among other factors, are also key influences. Moreover, gender norms are constructed and learned differently in different settings, and it is important that we keep in mind this cultural variability even as we discuss common tendencies in how norms shape the sexual vulnerability and health of young women and young men. Although prescribed norms in terms of gender roles and sexuality for women and for men seem to be nearly universal in some aspects, cultural differences would suggest that making universal conclusions about this body of research would be imprudent. To give just one example, young women have nearly equal sexual 'freedom' – that is, freedom to have sexual relations before marriage or outside stable unions – in some parts of the world and in some cultural groups, while there is a rigidity of separation of the sexes and enforcement of differences between males and females in other contexts (and of course major differences within these settings). What is fairly consistent in most developing country settings and many industrialised settings is the sex-specific segregation of boys and girls. Time-use studies in many settings find that boys spend more of their time outside the home, while girls are more likely to stay in or around the home – what some researchers have called a 'culture of the street', or external sphere for boys, and a 'culture of the bedroom' or the house for girls (Emler and Reicher, 1995; Mensch *et al.*, 1998).

Similarly, we must also keep in mind the variability of gender norms across history. As we have tried to emphasise, gender norms are complex and dynamic across cultural and historical realities and, in contemporary times, there have been many notable transformations in gender roles, particularly for young women. For example, one of the most cited gains in the movement for gender-equity has been the increased participation of women in the labour force. In many urban, Western contexts (and some other contexts as well) there has been increased attention to expanding opportunities for young women, and even a loosely defined movement around 'girl power' and the new femininities associated with it. Indeed, there is evidence that girls and women are finding new voices and new spaces (in the world of sports, in positions of leadership, in universities, and in other settings) with implications (generally positive) for their sexual and reproductive health and opportunities. These changes provide examples of the dynamic nature of gender, and further highlight the need to avoid painting a picture of women and girls as merely powerless victims of male oppression or patriarchy.

Another point of complexity is the variability across individuals. As previously mentioned, gender is not an amorphous force, but rather an interaction of the many levels of the ecological model, such that individuals can reconstruct norms and can influence socio-cultural norms, even as they are shaped by them. It is also important to highlight that the ways by which individuals internalise gender norms are neither simple nor automatic; individuals are not empty vessels who are 'filled up' with external social norms. Gender role development consists of a dynamic process involving continuous construction and reconstruction of gender-related attitudes, values and behaviours.

Furthermore, ideas and attitudes about gender-related issues change over the course of the lifecycle, as well as across different life circumstances and different relationships. For example, girls and boys are raised and viewed differently from birth, but it is generally from puberty onward that the gender divide becomes more pronounced in terms of expectations, opportunities and behaviours (Mensch et al., 1998; UNFPA, 2005). From a developmental perspective, 'adolescence' can be seen as a period in which gender role differentiation often intensifies, and attitudes, behaviours and hierarchies of power in intimate and sexual relationships are rehearsed (Mensch et al., 1998; Barker et al., 2004). Again, while these are common patterns, individuals vary widely, change over time (in ways that may follow normative patterns but may also defy them) and bring, as we will describe below, a tremendous degree of subjectivity to the extent to which they may adhere to extant gender norms.

Structural factors

Among the various structural and community factors that have important implications for gender-specific vulnerabilities, there has been most discussion about access to and/or lack of socio-economic opportunities, health services, and social policies.

For young people, economic disempowerment has important implications for their sexual behaviour. For example, an ethnographic study in an Eastern Cape township in South Africa suggested that the lack of economic and recreational opportunities for youth led to sexual relations being used as a means of gaining respect and social status (Wood and Jewkes, 2001). It is also important to note that, while poverty has a negative influence on the health and behaviour of all young people, its impact is greater on young women who, in general, have less access to information and less negotiating power to influence decisions, including protecting themselves from HIV. Research has shown that the economic vulnerability of women makes it more likely that they will exchange sex for money or favours, less likely that they will succeed in negotiating protection, less likely that they will leave a relationship that they perceive to be risky, and less likely that they will be able to access formal support services (Heise and Elias, 1995; Weiss and Gupta, 1998).

In turn, for low-income young men who often lack other means of affirming their identity, being without work and income is not merely a question of poverty, unemployment, or underemployment, but it can also be an affront to their very sense of self. Work is how they define who they are in their social settings. Young women in these same settings may find meaningful, albeit limited, social roles and a sense of self as mothers or partners of men, but young men rarely find a socially recognised identity through carrying out domestic chores or caring for children. For most young and adult men, work is the chief basis of their identity, or the main cultural and personal requisite for achieving 'manhood'. For a young man, being able to financially support himself and his family is generally a precursor to reproduction. Thus, achieving the provider role (that is, acquiring gainful employment) may be a signal event for many young males to begin reproduction. For other males, having an unplanned child may be an impetus to acquire employment. For the most part, however, there is limited research on the links between young males' education, employment, and reproduction indicating a need for additional research and programmatic attention to this topic.

In some settings in parts of Latin America and the Caribbean, North America and Western Europe, and even in a few settings in Africa, the gender gap at the level of primary education has been narrowed and we begin to see gendered vulnerabilities of young men and boys; these include difficulties in staying focused on task, being socialised around a street-oriented version of manhood (as opposed to an academic-version of manhood), aggressive behaviour and school performance issues. In these settings, young men (particularly low income, urban-based young men and boys) are dropping out or leaving school at rates higher than young women, a trend which has implications for their access to information and services related to sexual health (WHO, 2000).

Another important structural factor related to the vulnerability of young women and young men is access to information and services. In many settings, information and resources related to sexuality and reproductive health are taboo, particularly in relation to adolescents. A recent (as yet unpublished) operations research study in public health clinics in Rio de Janeiro, coordinated by Instituto Promundo and PAHO, concluded that a lack of facilities with adequately trained health care professionals inhibited young people's use of health care (unpublished report, 2005). Similarly, scant informational materials for young people about sexuality and self-care signalled health care professionals' lack of readiness to work with young men and women.

In addition to the taboos and lack of resources to deal with young men's and women's reproductive health and sexuality, reproductive health is often seen as a 'female' concern and cultural norms might restrict the possibility for men to be involved in their partners' health or to voice concerns about their own health. Findings suggest that boys in many settings (North America, parts of Europe, Latin America and parts of sub-Saharan Africa) may delay seeking help longer than women and girls and may only seek help when the need has already led to significant personal consequences (Kutcher et al., 1996). This might be partially attributed to traditional gender norms that perpetuate ideals of risk and self-reliance, such that young men may have hesitations about seeking health services. In turn, public health workers may perceive that young men are disinterested and direct their efforts primarily to women (WHO, 2000).

Girls and young women, on the other hand, are more likely to use social support systems and pay attention to health-related issues and use health services (Frydenberg, 1997). However, in some settings, including parts of South Asia, the Middle East and parts of Africa, particularly northern Africa and rural areas, the ability of young women to access health services is limited by their relative lack of mobility. Other studies suggest that gender norms – along with age hierarchies, and taboos related to sexuality or other health issues, such as suicidal ideation or substance use – affect the nature of trust between young people and adults, and whether or not a young person turns to a parent or other adult, including health providers, for help (WHO, 1997).

Services are but one component of promoting sexual and reproductive health amongst young people. Various studies have confirmed that, while offering 'youth friendly' services is a vital component of any integrated and holistic public health system, simply offering quality and youth-friendly services will not promote health-seeking behaviours. Operations research by WHO and others confirms that most young people need information, counselling, and the ability to question rigid gender norms (and other rigid social norms) probably more so than they need health services (WHO, 2002). Clearly, some young people have a need for more and better health services, and health professionals often lack the skills and attitudes to work with young people in sensitive ways. But research would suggest that services are not the panacea for the sexual and reproductive health needs of young people and that community and peer spaces seem to be the most influential and effective in reaching youth, particularly in terms of promoting changes in norms around sexual behaviours (FOCUS, 2001; WHO, 2002).

Many of the contextual factors discussed thus far raise important policy issues linked to the vulnerability of young women and young men, including poverty, violence, education and discrimination. It is important, for example, that policies should actively promote the dissemination of information and access to services to promote the sexual and reproductive health of young people, as well as attempting to combat underlying societal inequities that can hinder young people's access to information and important social service supports. The promotion and protection of education can both have direct positive impacts on the lives of young men and young women as well as broader effects on the socio-cultural norms that might define their vulnerability. In a similar vein, education can also be a channel for teaching and reinforcing gender-equitable norms and attitudes.

Interpersonal relationships

At the interpersonal level, family, peers and partners play a substantial role in the development of gender-related attitudes and sexual behaviours. Across settings, family is usually the primary or most proximal social institution within which gender norms and roles are learned and reinforced. In particular, parents and relatives have a profound influence on the differentiated development of sexual behaviours among young men and young women. The most proximal and influential models for marital and parental roles in a young person's life are often the practices he or she witnesses within his or her own family. In a qualitative study conducted in Rio de Janeiro, a common factor among young men who demonstrated gender-equitable attitudes was the presence of nurturing male role models in their family or extended family setting (Barker, 2000). Female family members also have an important role in influencing how young men understand gender roles in the manner that they either reinforce or challenge traditional gender norms. For young women, families and societies may often restrict their access to information about sex or discourage related discussions out of fear that these might encourage sexual activity (Vasconcelos *et al.*, 1997; Petchesky and Judd, 1998). By contrast, young men are expected to be knowledgeable, aggressive, and experienced regarding sexuality and reproductive health issues (WHO, 2000).

In addition to the family, peer groups become increasingly influential with age in the construction and questioning of gender roles and development of attitudes, knowledge and behaviours of young men and young women, including sexual behaviour. In a developmental framework, these are the years when young men are socially pressured to gain autonomy from their parents (WHO, 2000). Often, peers will become the primary source for information on issues related to sex and sexuality, and particularly young men's perceptions of risky sexual behaviours (Moore and Rosenthal, 1993). Peer groups can also function as protective forces in the development of young men and young women. For young men who may not have male figures within their families, peers can serve as positive role models (WHO, 2000). Also, as young men progressively gain more autonomy from their families, peer groups provide an important social network within which they can seek support and a sense of belonging (WHO, 2000). For young women, peer environment plays an important role in the decision to use condoms. Young women in stable relationships are likely to be influenced by their girlfriends' decisions to use condoms or to engage in risky sexual behaviour (Norris and Ford, 1998). Similarly, for young men, believing that one's male peers use condoms has been found to be associated with higher levels of reported condom use (WHO, 2000).

In intimate relationships, gender roles are inextricably linked to interpersonal power dynamics, and gender-based power dynamics have important implications for the sexual behaviour and vulnerability of both women and men. Research in the USA and South Africa, for example, has found that women who perceive that they have less power in their romantic relationships are less likely to be able to negotiate safer sexual practices, and are more likely to be HIV positive (Pulerwitz et al., 2002; Pettifor et al., 2004). Similarly, women's perceptions of higher power in their intimate relationships have been linked to higher self-efficacy about using condoms and more positive expectancies of condom use (Soet et al., 1999). In the wake of the HIV epidemic, there has been increasing attention to women's economic dependency on men and its power-related implication for contexts such as marriage, and in transactional sex.

Individual factors

Around the time of puberty, individuals acquire more complex cognitive abilities, including the capacity for abstract thinking. This can lead to a questioning of gender norms, such that, while socio-cultural norms, structural factors and inter-personal relations have a definite weight on sexual behaviour, the individual also has the capacity to reflect on the potential to act in ways counter to prevailing gender norms. As discussed above, individuals are not empty vessels for the passive reception of gender norms or social norms of any kind; rather, they have the capacity to develop their own gender consciousness, or critical attitudes about gender norms. Moreover, they can develop the belief in their ability to act (self-efficacy) in more gender-equitable or gender-empowered ways than prevalent social norms might generally suggest. In this way, while young people may be vulnerable because of a series of social and structural factors, they can also reflect about gender norms critically and alter their own behaviour and the institutions around them through collective action. Gender-consciousness, as we use the term here, is an individual factor that refers to how individuals act on, question or live out gender norms in their social setting.

The concept of 'gender consciousness' originates from the idea of critical consciousness first developed by Paulo Freire. The process of 'conscientisation', according to Freire, links to the capacity of individuals to reflect on the world and to choose a given course of future action (Blackburn, 2000). This process of reflecting critically on the history of cultural conditions and class structures that support and frame experiences of gender inequality can help to promote personal growth, political awareness and activism that can create the conditions to change gender role prescriptions. In short, gender consciousness, through a process of critical reflection, can empower individuals to believe in their ability to act in more gender-equitable ways, or in other words, to develop a high sense of self-efficacy.

At the risk of oversimplifying what is a complex social phenomenon, there is a relevant metaphor in Matrix, the 1999 movie by Andy and Larry Wachowski. In this film, most of the characters live their lives unaware that all of their experiences and actions are constructs of a computer programme. Pursuing the metaphor, we can argue that gender norms form a matrix that influences human relationships and interactions, and which for many persons is unperceived. Most young women and men can perceive, and tell us about, the social pressures to act and behave in certain ways. But most young women and men do not have the ability to see beyond the matrix or to see the gender matrix for what it truly is – a socially constructed set of mandates shaped and created by individuals, social structures and historical and local contexts.

In the case of young men, we need to consider their ability to question idealised norms around manhood (particularly within their peer group) and, for young women, the ability to question norms that make them subservient. We also need to work with young men to enable them to have 'voice' to question traditional norms and to give 'voice' to the numerous existing individuals (perhaps even a majority in some settings) who already question gender inequities but do not feel empowered to state this or show this publicly. Although we cannot affirm that critical attitudes about gender norms automatically lead individuals to develop increased self-efficacy and/or engage in healthy sexual relationships, raising one's awareness about gender equity (and about existing inequities), and encouraging reflection about one's ability to act upon more equitable gender norms, are fundamental prerequisites.

Self-efficacy has long been identified as a key factor in reducing vulnerabilities for sexual and reproductive health (Bandura, 1977; Mantell *et al.*,

1997). Studies on sexuality have mostly focused on self-efficacy only in the realm of sexual behaviour, but it is important to note that the confidence in one's ability to act in other domains, including mobility and management of financial resources, also has important implications for sexual behaviours. While clearly related to the internalisation of gender norms, self-efficacy is also affected by other realms of an individual's life, such as educational attainment and employment, as well as the nature of a relationship.

Many studies have shown that self-efficacy is a complex multi-faceted concept, and that gender differences in the belief in one's ability to act vary strongly across cultures (Parsons *et al.*, 2000; Soler *et al.*, 2000). However, while there have been studies analysing the links between self-efficacy and specific sexual and reproductive health indicators, such as condom use, there is less known about gender differences in self-efficacy (Meekers and Klein, 2002). The research that does exist, particularly relating to condom use, has reinforced the links between traditional gender norms and power dynamics and self-efficacy. For example, a study with young people in urban Cameroon found that young women were significantly less likely than young men to believe that they can actually convince their partner to use condoms (Meekers and Klein, 2002). Moreover, women who lacked confidence in their ability to purchase condoms and negotiate their use tended to have a higher likelihood of engaging in unprotected intercourse, pointing to the default power men usually hold in the negotiation of sexual relations and condom use.

We want to be careful, however, not to overstate the potential or power of individuals to question or change social norms (see also the chapter by Ingham in this same volume). For both young men and young women, questioning gender norms also requires changes at the external or structural level. A young woman in Pakistan, with limited freedom to move outside her home, for example, may have limited 'space' to question social norms. That is, she may question them and abhor them but have limited instrumental ability to act on her questioning. In such settings, increasing young women's self-efficacy and assertiveness can run the risk of causing friction with parents and families. This conflict can arise in more traditional settings as well as in cases such as immigrant families from Central America and Mexico in the USA, or South Asian immigrant families in the UK, where traditional cultural values might clash with newer ideas about young women's rights (Tohid, 2003; Hondagneu-Sotelo, 2005).

Integrating gender positively in programme development

Using the ecological model, we have sought to demonstrate how structural and social 'sources' of gender norms interact with individuals, who have significant but not unlimited ability to question, criticise and reshape norms. At the nexus of this interaction between the individual and their social context, we have argued for the importance of gender consciousness and self-efficacy. We have also sought to highlight the limitations of this model for explaining the complexity of individual young people in diverse and dynamic contexts.

As mentioned in the introduction, there has been an increasing consensus in the last two decades on the need to integrate gender into programming. To a lesser degree, there has also been increasing evidence on the effectiveness of specific approaches. Building upon our discussion of gender within the context of the ecological model, we would like to highlight those approaches that most closely apply to what has been called 'gender transformative' programming, that is, programming that seeks to challenge rigid gender norms and relations and promote women's empowerment and male involvement (Gupta 2000; Gupta *et al.*, 2002). As gender norms and gender-related attitudes and behaviours are complex constructs that represent an interplay of socio-cultural, structural, community, interpersonal and individual factors, programming should address these various 'ecological' factors broadly and simultaneously. Emerging lessons from such programmes that have explicitly addressed gender with such a ecological perspective point to the importance of (i) promoting critical reflections of gender and socialisation in educational activities, (ii) the creation of environments in which individual and group-level changes are supported by changes in social norms and institutions and (iii) broader alliance-building across Government, civil society and local communities to contribute to and reinforce positive changes in norms around gender and sexuality.

Critical reflections of gender and socialisation

Research and programme findings suggest that the binomial of internalised gender norms and self-efficacy is key to understanding how gender relates to the sexual behaviour and vulnerabilities of young people. Thus, at the individual level, it is important to promote both men's and women's gender consciousness and help them develop skills so they can feel more capable of acting in more gender-equitable and empowered ways, including the ability to negotiate with partners, question peer groups and seek services.

A handful of concrete and deliberate efforts in different parts of the world have demonstrated measurable changes in attitudes and behaviours among young people as a result of including discussions of gender norms and socialisation in educational activities. These efforts include the *Girls Power Initiative* in Nigeria (Irvin, 2000), *Men as Partners* in South Africa (Mehta *et al.*, 2004), *Program H* in Latin America (Barker et al, 2004) and *Stepping Stones* (White *et al.*, 2003), originally developed in Uganda but now implemented regionally. Moreover, these programmes, among others, have shown that the workshop format provides the best example of dynamic discussion spaces in which individuals can reflect critically and build gender consciousness, as well as 'rehearse' the skills and abilities necessary to act in more equitable and/or empowered ways (Gupta, 2002; Barker *et al.*, 2004).

In the case of the *Program H* and *Men As Partners* programmes, these discussions are systematised in curricula, which are made available to partner organisations, who in turn can incorporate gender reflections into their own activities. It is important to emphasise that these discussions about gender norms and relations are not simply 'feel-good' discussion groups or group therapy. Rather, they are concrete and deliberate efforts to engage young women and young men in critical analyses of gender roles which, when adequately structured, can lead to measurable changes in attitudes and behaviours.

Creating enabling environments

In addition to working with small groups of young men and young women, it is important to also seek to change the social environment and engage peer groups, social groups, and entire communities in the questioning, criticism and reconstruction of norms related to gender and sexual and reproductive health. *Puntos de Encuentro* in Nicaragua (White *et al.*, 2003) and *Soul City* in South Africa (White *et al.*, op. cit.) use multimedia strategies, including radio and television, to generate debate amongst diverse groups of viewers and to foster enabling environments for cultural change, especially related to gender and sexuality norms, stigma, and social support systems.

Broader alliance building

Changing gender norms is a slow process, and the reality is that without active government and civil society commitment through legislative, administrative, and financial means, there can be few profound changes in gender norms or the other contextual factors linked to the vulnerabilities of young women and young men. Therefore, initiatives on a large scale will only be as effective as such efforts to eradicate negative social and economic factors, including gender, racial, and socio-economic inequalities. In response, many programmes have sought to additionally build broad-based alliances with Government and civil society at the local and sometimes national level to promote more equitable policy and social environments. In this way, messages offered through group educational activities, community campaigns, educational materials, and social service settings can be echoed and reinforced at several levels.

Conclusions

Factoring gender into sexual health programming means moving beyond simplistic intervention models of information or service provision.

Instead, programmes should include critical discussions of norms and provide spaces in which young men and young women can build skills that allow them to act in more equitable and/or empowered ways. Similarly, it is not enough to only offer services but, rather, programmes should also work to change attitudes around gender-related norms of the providers offering them. Furthermore, while individuals are capable of challenging rigid norms, we cannot expect that merely teaching young people to question norms is sufficient, particularly if they have no objective means – freedom of movement, access to services – to do so. It is important to also carry out more broad-reaching efforts, from community-level mobilisation to advocacy, to overcome structural and other environmental factors that create gender-related vulnerabilities for young men and young women.

Above all, however, the challenge lies in tapping into the voices of resistance and change that exist in diverse contexts– those young men and young women who demonstrate and advocate more equitable and more empowered ways of living together. Ultimately, it will be these voices that will promote the necessary individual, community and social changes.

Acknowledgements

The authors would like to offer special thanks to Hena Khan of Horizons and Marcos Nascimento and Luciana Rodrigues, both of Instituto Promundo, for their valuable help with comments and editing.

References

Bandura. A. (1977) Self-efficacy: Toward a unifying theory of behavioural change, *Psychological Review*, 84(2), 191–215.

Barker, G. (2000) Gender equitable boys in a gender inequitable world: Reflections from qualitative research and program development in Rio de Janeiro, *Sexual and Relationship Therapy*, 15(3), 263–282.

Barker, G., Nascimento, M., Segundo, M., and Pulerwitz, J. (2004) How do we know if men have changed? Promoting and measuring attitude change with young men: Lessons from Program H in Latin America, in S. Ruxton (ed.) *Gender Equality and Men: Learning from practice*, Oxford: Oxfam GB, 147–61.

Blackburn, J. (2000) Understanding Paulo Freire: Reflections on the origins, concepts, and possible pitfalls of his educational approach, *Community Development Journal*, 35(1), 3–15.

Boender, C., Santana, D., Santillán, D., Hardee, K., Greene, M. and Schuler, S. (2004) *The 'So What' Report: A look at whether integrating a gender focus into programs makes a difference to outcomes*, Washington DC: Interagency Gender Working Group Task Force.

Bronfenbrenner, U. (1979) *The Ecology of Human Development: Experiments by nature and design*, Cambridge, MA: Harvard University Press.

Eggleston, J. and Hardee, K. (1999) Sexual attitudes and behaviour among young adolescents in Jamaica, *International Family Planning Perspectives*, 25, 78–84.

Emler, N. and Reicher, S. (1995) *Adolescence and Delinquency: The Collective Management of Reputation*, Oxford: Blackwell Publishers.

FOCUS (2001) *Advancing Young Adult Reproductive Health: Actions for the next decade*, Washington DC: Pathfinder International.

Frydenberg, E. (1997) *Adolescent Coping: Theoretical and Research Perspectives*, London: Routledge.

Gupta, G.R. (2000) Gender sexuality and HIV/AIDS: The what, the why and the how, plenary address at XIIIth. International AIDS Conference, Durban, South Africa, July 12, 2000.

Gupta, G.R., Whelan, D. and Allendorf, K. (2002) *Integrating Gender into HIV/AIDS Programs: Review paper for expert consultation*, 3–5 June 2002, Geneva: World Health Organisation.

Harrison, A., Xaba, N., and Kunene, P. (2001) Understanding safe sex: Gender narratives of HIV and pregnancy prevention by rural south African school-going youth, *Reproductive Health Matters*, 17, 63–71.

Heise, L. (1998) Violence against women: An integrated, ecological framework, *Violence Against Women*, 4(3), 262–90.

Heise, L. and Elias, C. (1995) Transforming AIDS prevention to meet women's needs: A focus on developing countries, *Social Science and Medicine*, 40(7), 933–43.

Heise, L., Ellsberg, M. and Gottemoeller, M. (1999) Ending violence against women, Population Reports, Series L, No. 11. Baltimore, Maryland: Johns Hopkins University School of Public Health, Center for Communications Programs, Population Information Program.

Hondagneu-Sotelo, P. (2005) *Gendering Migration: Not for 'feminists only' – and not only in the household*, CMD Working Paper #05–02f, Los Angeles, CA: University of Southern California.

Irvin, A. (2000) *Taking Steps of Courage: Teaching adolescents about sexuality and gender in Nigeria and Cameroon*, New York: International Women's Health Coalition.

Jejeebhoy, S.J. and Bott, S. (2003) *Non-consensual Sexual Experiences of Young People: A review of the evidence from developing countries*, New Delhi, India: Population Council.

Khan, M.E., Khan, I. and Mukerjee, N. (1998) Men's attitude towards sexuality and their sexual behaviour: Observations from rural Gujarat, paper presented at the seminar on Men, Family Formation and Reproduction, Buenos Aires, Argentina, May 13–15, 1998.

Kutcher, S., Ward, B., Hayes, D., Wheeler, K., Brown, F., and Kutcher, J. (1996) Mental health concerns of Canadian adolescents: A consumer's perspective, *Canadian Journal of Psychiatry*, 41(1), 5–10.

Mantell, J.E., DiVittis, A.T. and Auerbach, M.I. (1997) *Evaluating HIV Prevention Programs*, New York: Plenum Press.

Marsiglio, W. (1988) Adolescent male sexuality and heterosexual masculinity: A conceptual model and review, *Journal of Adolescent Research*, 3(3–4), 285–303.

McLeroy, K.R., Bibeau, D., Steckler, A. and Glanz, K. (1988) An ecological perspective on health promotion programs, *Health Education Quarterly*, 15(4), 351–77.

Meekers, D. and Klein, M. (2002) Understanding gender differences in condom use self-efficacy among youth in urban Cameroon, *AIDS Education and Prevention*, 14(1), 62–72.

Mehta, M., Peacock, D. and Bernal, L. (2004) Men as partners: Lessons learned from engaging men in clinics and communities, in S. Ruxton (ed.) *Gender Equality and Men: Learning from practice*, Oxford: Oxfam GB, 89–100.

Mensch, B., Bruce, J. and Greene, M.E. (1998) *The Uncharted Passage: Girls' adolescence in the developing world*. New York: Population Council.

Moore, S., and Rosenthal, D. (1993) *Sexuality in Adolescence*. London: Routledge.

Norris, A.E. and Ford, K. (1998) Moderating influence of peer norms on gender differences in condom use, *Applied Developmental Science*, 2(4), 174–81.

Nzioka, C. (2001) Perspectives of adolescent boys on the risks of unwanted pregnancy and sexually transmitted infections: Kenya, *Reproductive Health Matters*, 9,108–117.

Parsons, J., Halkitis, P., Bimbi, D. and Borkowshi, T. (2000) Perceptions of the benefits and costs associated with condom use and unprotected sex among late adolescent college students, *Journal of Adolescence*, 23(4), 377–91.

Petchesky, R.P. and Judd, K. (eds) (1998) *Negotiating Reproductive Rights: Women's perspectives across countries and cultures*, New York: Zed Books Ltd.

Pettifor, A.E., Measham, D.M., Rees, H.V. and Padian, N.S. (2004) Sexual power and HIV risk, South Africa, *Emerging Infectious Diseases* (available online at <www.cdc.gov/ncidod/EID/vol10no11/04–0252.htm>).

Pulerwitz, J., Amaro, H., De Jong, W., Gortmaker, S.L. and Rudd, R. (2002) Relationship power, condom use and HIV risk among women in the USA, *AIDS Care*, 14, 789–800.

Rivers, K. and Aggleton, P. (1999) *Adolescent Sexuality, Gender and the HIV Epidemic*, New York: United Nations Development Programme.

Rogers, E. (1995) *Diffusion of Innovations, 4th edition*, New York, NY: The Free Press.

Sallis, J.F. and Owen, N. (2002) Ecological models of health behaviour, in K. Glanz, B.K. Rimer and F.M. Lewis (eds) *Health Behaviour and Health Education: Theory, research and practice,* 3rd edition, San Francisco: Jossey-Bass Publishers, 462–84.

Schueller, J., Finger, W. and Barker, G. (2005) *Boys and Changing Gender Roles: Emerging program approaches hold promise in changing gender norms and behaviours among boys and young men*, Washington, DC: Youth Net.

Soet, J. E., Dudley, W. N., and DiIorio, C. (1999) The effects of ethnicity and perceived power on women's sexual behaviour, *Psychology of Women Quarterly*, 23, 707–23.

Soler, H., Quadagno, D., Sly, D., Riehman, K., Eberstein, I., and Harrison, D. (2000) Relationship dynamics, ethnicity and condom use among low-income women, *Family Planning Perspectives*, 32(2), 82–8, 101.

Tohid, O. (2003) Pakistanis abroad trick daughters into marriage, *The Christian Science Monitor*, May 15, 2003 (available online at <www.csmonitor.com/2003/0515/p01s03-wosc.htm>).

UN (1995) *Report of the Fourth World Conference on Women, Beijing*, 4–15 September 1995, New York: United Nations.

UNFPA (1994) *Program of Action of the International Conference on Population and Development,* Cairo, 5–13 September 1994 (available online at <http://www.unfpa.org/icpd/icpd_poa.htm>).

UNFPA (2000) *Partnering: A new approach to sexual and reproductive health,* Technical Paper, No.3, New York: UNFPA.

UNFPA (2005) *State of the World Population: The promise of equality gender equity, reproductive health and the millennium development goals,* New York: UNFPA.

Varga, C. (2003) How gender roles influence sexual and reproductive health among South African adolescents, *Studies in Family Planning,* 34(3), 160–72.

Vasconcelos, A., Garcia, V., Mendonca, M. C., Pacheco, M., das Gracas Braga Pires, M., Tassitano, C. and Garcia, C. (1997) *Sexuality and AIDS prevention among adolescents in Recife, Brazil,* Washington DC: International Center for Research on Women, Women and AIDS Research Program.

Weiss, E. and Gupta, G.R. (1998) *Bridging the Gap: Addressing Gender and Sexuality in HIV Prevention,* Washington, DC: International Center for Research on Women.

White, V., Greene, M. and Murphy, E. (2003) *Men and Reproductive Health Programs: Changing gender norms,* Washington DC: The Synergy Project.

WHO (1997) *Young People and their Families: A cross cultural study of parent/adolescent discord in Cote d'Ivoire, India and Nigeria,* Geneva: World Health Organisation.

WHO (2000) *What About Boys? A Literature Review on the Health and Development of Adolescent Boys,* Geneva: World Health Organisation and Pan American Health Organisation.

WHO (2002) *Global Consultation on Adolescent Friendly Health Services: A presentation of consensus statements, the basis of these statements, and their implications for research and action: Working Draft,* 7–9 March 2001, Geneva: World Health Organisation.

Wood, K. and Jewkes, R. (2001) Dangerous Love: Reflections on violence among Xhosa Township youth, in R. Morell (ed.) *Changing Men in Southern Africa,* Pietermaritzburg: University of Natal Press.

Part 2

Chapter 5

Meeting the sexual health needs of young people living on the street

Elaine Chase and Peter Aggleton

Introduction

Across the world, some tens of millions of children and young people live on the street (UNICEF, 2006). Although precise numbers are difficult to assess, global population growth and wordwide urbanisation, alongside other social, economic and environmental factors, have inevitably meant a steady increase in their number. In more recent years, and particularly since the onset of the global HIV pandemic, there has been a growing interest in the sexual and reproductive health and wellbeing of homeless children and young people and how best to mitigate the many factors that may increase their vulnerability to poor sexual health outcomes.

Children and young people may find themselves homeless for a variety of reasons. HIV/AIDS (Ansell and van Blerk, 2004; Ansell and Young, 2004), war and political turmoil (Mann, 2004), drought, famine and economic crisis (Ochola, 2000), have all been cited as factors affecting young people's movement onto the streets. Other individual factors range from abuse and neglect on the one hand, to the search for economic freedom on the other (Barker and Knaul, 2000; Kudrati *et al.*, 2002). While negative 'push' factors such as war, poverty and abuse may render many young people homeless, others are drawn to street life by 'pull' factors such as following friends, desiring drugs, or opportunities to earn money (*Casa de Passagem*, 1997, quoted in Barker and Knaul, 2000; Kudrati *et al.*, 2002).

Once on the street, young people lose contact with their families and communities of origin to differing extents (Swart-Kruger and Richter, 1997; Ochola, 2000; Barker and Knaul, 2000). As a result, they may lose access to both formal programmes providing information and services to promote their sexual health, and to some of the informal networks from which they can learn about protective cultural norms and values governing sex and sexuality. Although young people living on the street are likely to have complex sexual and reproductive health needs, surprisingly little has been documented about them, and the evidence-base for the types of programmatic responses that might best respond to these needs is weak.

In this chapter, the situations faced by children and young people on the street are discussed alongside the risks to their sexual health. The available literature concerning the sexual health of street-living young people is described alongside findings from some recently conducted research among street-living young people in Zimbabwe. As such, the chapter explores how factors identified in the broader literature intersect and affect real lives. While recognising that living on the street presents profound and indisputable challenges to young people's sexual health and wider wellbeing, the chapter discusses the importance of approaches to sexual health promotion that are both meaningful and contextualised within young people's life circumstances. It discusses the inadequacies of viewing street living young people solely through a lens that focuses on their passivity, victimisation and their need for protection. Such an approach risks both misrepresenting the challenges that these young people face and undermining their collective capacity to define their own responses. Rather, we argue that programme responses which strike a balance between acknowledging street-living young people's vulnerability and enabling them to take greater control over factors affecting their sexual health are more likely to have a positive impact on their wellbeing.

Who are street-living children and young people?

A number of definitions of street children have emerged in the literature over the years and, while some differentiation is made between street children and street youth, the terms are frequently used interchangeably. In accordance with the definition of 'child' within the United Nations Convention on the Rights of the Child (UNCRC) (UNICEF, 1989), the term *street children* refers primarily in such literature to all children and young people under 18 years.

Probably the most commonly cited definition of street children is 'any girl or boy ... for whom the street (in the widest sense of the word, including unoccupied dwellings, wasteland, and so on) has become his or her habitual abode and/or source of livelihood; and who is inadequately protected, supervised, or directed by responsible adults (Inter-NGO definition, cited in Ennew, 1994, p.15). Most other definitions of street children encompass notions of abandonment, poverty and lack of adult supervision, support and protection (WHO, 2000; Marino, 2003). Yet such designations fall short of adequately describing the range of different circumstances and lifestyles of street living children and young people. Panter-Brick (2003) has identified serious inadequacies and difficulties with the commonly used term street children. These include its negativity, its failure to encompass the heterogeneity of street living children and young people and their movement on and off the street, and the fact that the term may be used to reflect particular contemporary social and political agendas (particularly those of donor agencies), often, as a result, deflecting attention away from many other children living in abject poverty.

Similarly, terms such as 'of the street' and 'on the street' used by UNICEF (2001) to differentiate between children and young people living and sleeping on the street or spending their day on the street and returning home at night, have been found to fall short of describing actual experiences. Some young people may sleep on the street for a period of time and then return home (Barker and Knaul, 2000; Panter-Brick, 2003); others spend some time in institutions or in police detention, or move between the houses of others, the street and institutions to meet their basic needs (Barker and Knaul, 2000; Raffaelli *et al.,* 2000). De Moura (2005) has described the multiple changes in social environment experienced by children on the street and illustrated how environments that street children pass through, such as institutions, substitute care, family homes and shelters, can be as transitional as their lives on the streets.

Ochola (2000) has identified at least four categories of children and young people living on the streets of African cities; those who continue to have contact with their families, those who lose family contact, those who live in 'gangs' in temporary makeshift shelters, and those who are living with parents on the street and are part of an increasing number of street families, with some of these parents being 'adolescents' themselves. In their work on street girls and young women, Barker and Knaul (2000) draw a distinction between street girls who have limited contact with their family, and working girls who work with or without other family members in exchange for cash or goods, either in open spaces (such as street markets) or in enclosed environments such as other people's homes. Swart-Kruger and Richter (1997) talk of young people experiencing varying degrees of dislocation from family, school and community, and who work, congregate and/or live in urban areas.

Overall, the proportion of children and young people actually living on the street, as opposed to working on the street, may be relatively small. Studies have also noted that the proportion of girls living on the street is far lower than that of boys (Swart-Kruger and Richter, 1997; Rurevo and Bourdillon, 2003; UNICEF, 2006). Barker and Knaul (1991), for example, have suggested that between 3 and 30 per cent of street-living children throughout the world are girls. However, the proportion of girls on the street is on the increase (Raffaelli *et al.,* 2000; WERK, 2002) and, although young women may be less prominent on the street than boys, there is evidence to suggest that it is harder for them to return home and that they are less likely to maintain links with family (Barker and Knaul, 2000; Raffaelli *et al.,* 2000; UNICEF, 2006).

Sexual health risks on the street

Much of what is written about the sexual health risks faced by girls and boys on the street is linked to the need (either occasional or regular) to engage in transactional or survival sex (see also Chapter 4 in this volume); that is, sex in exchange for money, food, shelter and other basic commodities. Both boys and girls may also secure protection from violence or mistreatment through having sex (WHO, 2000; Rurevo and Bourdillon, 2003). Young people on the street have less access than other young people to information about the risks of sexually transmitted infections, unplanned pregnancies or illegal abortions (Barker and Knaul, 2000; Rurevo and Bourdillon, 2003), and may be misinformed about behaviours that may and may not be hazardous to their sexual health (Raffaelli *et al.*, 1993; 1995; Swart-Kruger and Richter, 1997). They are also less likely to have access to condoms and contraceptive services and advice that enable them to reduce their vulnerability to poor sexual health outcomes (Barker and Knaul, 2000) and may hold negative attitudes towards condom use (Swart-Kruger and Richter, 1997).

There has been a tendency in the literature, however, to make broad generalisations about the risks encountered by street youth in regard to their sexual, as well as physical and mental, health. Such assumptions are made without fully investigating the nature of what constitutes risks in different circumstances and for different young people, and what processes enable children and young people to cope or negotiate these risks (Panter-Brick, 2003).

Rarely are distinctions made between coercive, exploitative or violent relationships and the romantic relationships (Swart-Kruger and Richter, 1997) that young people may enter into while living on the street. WHO (2000), for example, identifies four main types of sex which young people on the street are likely to have: *comfort sex,* to replace relationships or attachments with others; *sex for power,* or as a means of gaining or maintaining control over others; initiation sex, and *sex for punishment,* when young people do not conform to group norms or the rules of group or gang leaders. By contrast, Rajani and Kudrati (1996), in their work on the sexual experiences of street children in Mwanza, Tanzania, identified the fact that what outside observers frequently perceived as negative or coercive relationships between young people were, in fact, considered, particularly by girls, to be relationships based on love, physical attraction and friendship.

This said, the sexual health risks faced by young people on the street are often inextricably linked to their circumstances and their limited access to resources, a factor which may be more pronounced for girls and young women than for boys and young men. A number of studies in Zimbabwe (Rurevo and Bourdillon, 2003), Brazil (Swift, 1997), Zambia (Lopi and Kiremire, 2001) and Sudan (Kudrati *et al.*, 2002), have all shown that girls on the street have fewer opportunities than boys to make a living. As a result, they were most commonly found to be limited to petty vending, begging and exchanging sex for money or basic commodities.

To date, there is a limited literature on the circumstances surrounding the street life of girls on the street and the sexual health risks and difficulties they face (Wutoh *et al.*, 2002; Dybicz, 2005). Unwanted pregnancies, street abortions, STIs and HIV, as well as sexual abuse and violence, have all been identified as key sexual health problems faced by girls and young women living on the street (Raffaelli *et al.*, 1993; Barker and Knaul, 2000; Ruvero and Bourdillon, 2003). Girls have also reported commonly being stigmatised as prostitutes, a factor that commonly perpetuates a high degree of sexual violence towards them (Rurevo and Bourdillon, 2003). These sexual health risks are often exacerbated by the practical and psychological difficulties in accessing appropriate support and health services, including a lack of available health facilities and the negative attitudes of health workers (Barker and Knaul, 2000).

While girls and young women may face a wider range of negative consequences to their sexual health including unplanned pregnancy or illegal abortions, the specific risks for boys and young men may be less visible. There is evidence that many boys and young men exchange sex with both men and women for money, food, shelter or basic resources (Raffaelli *et al.*, 1993; 1995; Swart-Kruger and Richter, 1997). The degree of reciprocity within these relationships or the extent to which they are exploitative is poorly understood. Boys and young men who have same sex relationships with other men are likely to experience stigma and face difficulties in accessing services to promote their sexual health.

The combination of the broader societal and environmental factors that precipitate movement on to the street, the group or social networks they become a part of, and the lack of services and programmes designed to address their specific sexual health needs thus work together synergistically to increase young people's vulnerability to poor sexual health outcomes (Aggleton *et al.*, 2004).

Contextualising the risk to young people's sexual health – a case study

Despite the range of potential sexual health difficulties they may encounter, the risk of pregnancy or infection has been found to be a low priority for street-living young people compared to the need to secure money, food, clothes and shelter (Swart-Kruger and Richter, 1997) or to secure a regular supply of drugs (Inciardi and Surratt, 1997). Young people on the street are also frequently subjected to extensive discrimination and stigmatisation, including police detention or brutality (Inciardi and Surratt, 1997; Ochola, 2000). These factors create a particular challenge for sexual health programming and raise important questions about the types of approaches that may or may not be relevant. The following case study, drawn from recent work in Zimbabwe undertaken by the first author (Elaine Chase), illustrates some of the complex day to day circumstances for young people on the street and the types of approaches taken by a non-governmental organisation (NGO) to support them.

In January 2004, a qualitative in-depth study was undertaken commissioned by Catholic Relief Services (CRS) in Zimbabwe (Chase *et al.*, 2006). Using a combination of household case studies and semi-structured interviews with children in different circumstances, the study investigated the lives, needs and coping strategies of orphans and vulnerable children and young people and their families in six contrasting sites (both urban and rural). In one of the urban sites, some time was spent investigating the situations of children and young people on the street. Young people were accessed through the sports and outreach activities of the *Streets Ahead* project in Harare, (www.streetsahead.org.zw). This project, established in 1992, works with 500 or more children and young people at any one time, the large majority of whom are boys and young men.

Staff at *Streets Ahead* reported that, since 2000, a combination of economic and social factors has caused a rapid increase in the numbers of children and young people living on the streets of Harare. As elsewhere in Southern Africa, HIV and AIDS have become key 'push' factors in bringing young people onto the streets. As an increasing number of adults become ill or die as a result of AIDS, it may no longer be possible for children who are orphaned to be absorbed in to fragile extended family networks (Baylies, 2002). At the end of 2003, there were an estimated 1,300,000 orphans in Zimbabwe, with 78 per cent (980,000) of these children having been orphaned as a result of HIV-related illness (UNAIDS/UNICEF/USAID, 2004).

A worsening economic climate and difficulties in securing a subsistence living in rural areas was cited by NGO staff as a key reason for the increasing numbers of children coming onto the streets of Harare. Young people were also reportedly being forced to leave their rural homes following accusations that they supported the party in opposition to the ruling Zanu PF party, or due to the knock-on effect of Government land resettlement programmes and the consequent displacement of farm labourers and their families. An increasing number of children have also arrived on the streets of Harare as part of a growing number of street-dwelling families.

Workers at *Streets Ahead* reported that the biggest problems for young people living on the street were a lack of washing facilities, a poor diet, unsafe sexual practices and substance use. The use of drugs, mainly glue and *ganja,* and alcohol make it very difficult to engage young people in education or skills training programmes. More than half of the young people that *Streets Ahead* work with reportedly sniff glue and/or drink Kachasu – alcohol traditionally made from wild fruits, but more recently distilled from fertiliser, soap, chemicals or any other substance available.

Streets Ahead offers a range of services to young people, some of which address their immediate needs, others the wider circumstances of their lives. These include outreach work and counselling, referral to other health and support services, and reunification with families and communities. The underlying philosophy is to work from what the children ask for and not to force a situation or set the agenda, since this latter approach runs the risk of the project team losing contact with the children and young people they are trying to help.

Both girls and boys on the streets of Harare were reported by project staff to be vulnerable to sexual exploitation through prostitution. Both women and men in the city were said to pay to have sex with young boys. The perception from staff was that these relationships between adults and children and young people were particularly exploitative, with very little money being paid to the young people.

In order to mitigate some of the sexual health risks faced by young people, the project increases access to diagnosis and treatment of sexually transmitted infections (STIs). On average, 25 young people each week are referred to a local doctor for treatment for sexually transmitted infections. Those who have concerns about HIV/AIDS, or who are HIV positive, are referred to local counselling and support services. For those who die on the street from HIV-related illnesses, accidents or other causes, the project pays for a coffin and food for those attending the funeral. A small group of peer leaders have been trained to introduce the project team to new children arriving on the street and to provide HIV and drugs prevention education. Peer group leaders are paid a small amount of money for this work.

The reunification work of the project involves counselling children and their families and relatives. The ethos of *Streets Ahead* is not to place children in institutions but to work with children and young people on the street. The organisation pays school fees and other school-related expenses for 70 children and runs a skills training centre where they teach dress making and carpentry. Children under 14 years old who are not able to cope with full-time education can access informal and part-time education facilities. The project works hard to try to secure birth certificates for children and young people since these are vital for them to access a range of support and education services.

The perceptions of project staff concerning key sexual health and drug issues were largely confirmed through observations and discussions with young people. The following examples, however, illustrate that, for street-dwelling young people, the need to sustain their lives and form meaningful social bonds with others on the street are likely to take precedence over concerns about their sexual health, a factor which has important implications for how sexual health projects and programmes are designed. All the names of young people have been changed and data were collected with guarantees of anonymity and informed consent.

John was 19-years-old and had been living on the street for eight months. Before then, he had lived in a children's home for four years. His father had died in 1997, followed by his mother in 2003. His older brother had left to live in South Africa and his three younger siblings lived in Chipinge with their grandmother.

John described how he spent his day on one particular street in town and slept at the bus terminus, on top of cardboard boxes, using sacks for blankets. In order to earn money, John looked after (stood guard for) or washed people's cars, carried people's luggage or did piece work such as carrying drinks to bars, or cleaning the passageways between shops. The work that he got dictated how many meals he could eat and he described how he frequently went for the whole day without eating. On a good day, however, he managed to eat in the morning, afternoon and evening. John slept at the bus terminus with about 14 other boys, some much younger than himself. He talked in detail about the frustration of people dropping their rubbish near where he slept and how he worried about the diseases he and the others could get from this lack of cleanliness such as 'malaria, cholera and stomach problems'.

John had been trained as a peer leader at his sleep and work bases and was involved in counselling and educating younger boys about the risks of sniffing glue. He said that sometimes the counselling worked and the boys 'leave it' (stopped taking it).

John then described how boys, 'both the older and younger ones', as well as girls were often taken away by 'rich' people from 'better places'. He talked of how they were given money in exchange for having sex with these people. They would be taken away from the streets for a time but would always come back. He did not know how much they were paid but said that they flashed money around when they returned. Both women and men were seen to take boys from the street. He commented that the boys who had sex with men did not talk to others about their experiences but knew each other well and tended to stay together – 'They say "this one is homosexual" and they don't to talk to the other guys on the street'. As far as he knew, the boys did not use any protection such as condoms when they had sex.

Chipo, aged 12, was originally from Bulawayo, a Ndebele speaking region of Zimbabwe, although he spoke perfect Shona. He first came to Harare with his mother (who has since returned to Bulawayo), and then ran away to live on the streets – 'I ran away and that's why I was not with Mum, I just enjoy living on the streets'. When asked to say more about his life before living on the streets, he revealed that his 'mother was a problem' and she used to beat him so he ran away. His father, he said, had died in 2001.

Chipo, like John, stayed at the bus terminus with his friends. He talked about having many friends, some older and some younger. He was wearing the only clothes that he possessed and had no shoes on his feet. Chipo commented that the girls spent time in different bases and he was 'not sure' what they did for money to survive. Chipo's main sources of income were begging and collecting and selling empty plastic containers to people who recycled them. He claimed that he ate three times a day and that when there was no money to buy food he picked food from the bins. Sometimes *Streets Ahead* provided them with food and, at other times, he and the other boys cooked together using empty cans for cooking and plastic to light the fire. When asked what foods he ate, Chipo said 'we eat sadza, sometimes rice ... whatever we can get in the bins'.

Chipo talked about his social relationships with others on the street. He described how there had previously been some 'horrible guys who were bullies' but that they had been arrested and, to his relief, no longer bothered him. He commented that the older boys protected him from those who were likely to bully him. When asked what he did all day, his response was 'sometimes it is so boring and sometimes it is so exciting. It is most exciting when we spend time together, tell each other stories and have fun together'.

Tatenda, 14-years-old, was really slight for his age. When we spoke to him he was wearing headphones connected to a small battered radio in his pocket and said he was listening to the news channel. He was wearing just one shoe, had very tattered clothes and was holding a plastic bottle with some glue in it. When asked about the glue, he said that one of the older boys had asked him to look after it.

Tatenda told us that after both of his parents had died, he had gone to stay with an aunt who had also died earlier that year (2004). Originally from a high density suburb outside Harare, he now slept on the street on cardboard boxes. He had five older sisters, all married and staying with their families. He did not stay with any of his sisters because their husbands did not want to keep him. Tatenda's main sources of income were looking after cars and begging. He frequently got food from the bins at the supermarket and often went for several days without eating. He talked about how he stayed with his 17-year-old cousin on the street. Although his cousin did not have any money to give him, he protected him. They had developed a reciprocal arrangement between themselves, whereby whoever got or earned money shared it with the other one. His biggest worry was about being arrested by police. He had witnessed some boys being beaten in custody and, although he had never been beaten himself, he had been detained overnight. When asked about the glue in his bottle, Tatenda said that most of the 'older guys' had glue which they sold to the younger boys by the lid-full from a plastic bottle. The boys sniffed glue, he thought, because 'they get drunk from it'.

Through the night outreach project of *Streets Ahead,* we met **Tafadzwa,** one of just three girls among a large group of 25–30 children and young people between the ages of nine and their late teens. The area they were congregated in was a work base and a sleep base for some of them, and just a work base for others. When the outreach team arrived, a dispute had broken out. The evident leader of the group, Kudzai, an older young man probably in his early twenties, claimed that the problem was that Tafadzwa, was 'having too many boyfriends' (having sex with different boys) and this was causing problems. The other girls present, friends of Tafadzwa, claimed that she was being forced to have sex with Kudzai. Others present confirmed that Kudzai wanted to control Tafadzwa and would not let her go anywhere without his permission.

Tafadzwa lived and slept on the street and had done so for about four months. Prior to that, she came onto the street only at weekends. She stayed together with one of the other girls in the group. Tafadzwa, who claimed that she was 20 years old, but thought by the project staff to be about 15 or 16, revealed that she was three months pregnant. She said that she had been feeling very tired and sick in pregnancy but that she had no money to attend a clinic. The *Streets Ahead* project worker explained that they would help her to see a doctor. Her friends and some of the boys present said that it would be better if the outreach team took Tafadzwa away with them as Kudzai would not allow her to see a doctor.

When the situation escalated, one of the project workers decided to take Tafadzwa off the street because she was not safe. At this point, Kudzai made a joke of offering $500 for her for sex. He became quite aggressive and wanted to be repaid for all the money that he said he had spent on food and drink for her. Tafadzwa appeared very frightened and agreed to leave with the project vehicle.

The observations made in this case study to a large extent accord with themes and issues highlighted in the literature described earlier. The case study has illustrated young people's preoccupation with securing a livelihood and the types of coping strategies they employ to access food and basic commodities. Also evident are the various factors that bring young people onto the street and the complex social relationships that develop between them once they are there. These have been documented to a greater or lesser extent elsewhere.

There are other instances, for example, of girls finding men to 'mind' them or aligning themselves to a protective gang of boys in exchange for sexual favours (Rurevo and Bourdillon, 2003). As Barker and Knaul (2000) have pointed out, 'non-normative' sexual behaviour is not necessarily sex work and girls who are sexually available to boys in a gang or group, or who trade sex for food and shelter, may be motivated by the need for security, identity and affection, rather than money.

Examples such as these illustrate not only young people's resourcefulness but also their ability to develop ways of negotiating situations so as to minimise some of the risks they face (Panter-Brick, 2003).

Recognising young people's social networks and social capital

Clearly evident in the case study above are the resourcefulness, reciprocity and mutual support that children and young people on the street gain from each other. These more creative and supportive aspects of street living have been largely downplayed in the published international literature. While it would be foolish to deny the reality of young people's more negative experiences, just as important is the fact that it is possible to harness the resourcefulness of young people and engage them in projects such as HIV and drug education with their younger peers.

Earlier in this chapter, we explored some of the language used to describe street children which defines their status in terms of the lack of protection and support awarded them by adults. Yet concepts of childhood, protection and care from adults vary enormously across different cultures and many children assume responsibilities similar to those of adults at a very young age (Boyden, 2003; Mann, 2004). While notions of 'neglect' fit with the constructs of childhood and parenting that have evolved in countries of Western Europe and North America, they may be less relevant (without careful adaptation) in other contexts. Most children and young people living on the streets of resource-poor countries, for example, are not brought up in ways that make them dependent on nuclear family structures for their social support and socialisation. Rather, wider extended family networks and the interdependence between these are more useful frameworks for understanding how separation from these can affect children (Mann, 2004). Even very young children in resource-poor communities are socialised to look after others, contribute to household and community economies and become self sufficient and independent of the family (Aptekar, 1991; Boyden, 2003; Mann, 2004). As a result, from an early age they learn the value of responsibility and cooperation and develop competencies outside of the experience of most European and North American children of similar ages.

Although children and young people living on the streets may become dislocated, to varying degrees, from established community social networks and their collective social capital, they are clearly able to form new social networks and generate their own social capital. This is both cognitive – feelings of a sense of community and perceptions of reciprocity, trust and shared values – and structural – participation in groupings or networks (Harpham, 2003). These forms of social capital created by young people themselves are not frequently recognised or understood (Harpham, 2003; Morrow, 2004).

Recent research among street children in Columbia has revealed the existence of complex social networks that serve an economic purpose by day and a social/ supportive purpose by night (Aptekar, 1991). Other research has demonstrated that young people on the street may replicate family structures and assume the roles of 'wives' and 'husbands' (Barker and Knaul, 2000). Significantly, as in families in other settings, these display both positive and negative characteristics. Ochola (2000) has described the intricate ties established between young people on the street and their frequent involvement in groups or gangs that have two key sets of functions;

maintenance, including providing an identity, support and relief from daily anxieties for group members, and task-orientated, directing income generating and survival activities. This same work has identified complex organisational structures and specialisation of activities by groups within distinct geographical boundaries to increase group effectiveness. An understanding of these mutually supportive networks between children and young people is likely the key to the design of sexual health programmes in street contexts.

Implications for future programmatic responses

Several themes emergent from both the literature and the research in Zimbabwe are relevant to the design and implementation of future programmes designed to promote the sexual and reproductive health needs of girls and boys living on the street.

First and foremost, programmes need to take account of the often complex reasons why young people end up on the street (Kudrati *et al.*, 2002). Girls and boys may have different motivating factors as to why they are on the street. Once the street becomes their source of livelihood, they may also have different ways of accessing available resources. On the whole, boys seem to have a wider range of economic opportunities than girls. A degree of gender differentiation is therefore required of health promotion initiatives which take account of the distinct circumstances of girls and boys and recognise that interventions that work for boys will not necessarily always be appropriate for work with girls. Gender may also combine with age to render young people more or less vulnerable in terms of their sexual and reproductive health (Swart-Kruger and Richter, 1997).

A careful analysis of the distinct life contexts of children and young people living on the street is required in designing appropriate sexual health programmes. These contexts vary widely across different parts of the world (Raffaelli et al, 2000; Ochola, 2000). Street-living young people experience diverse trajectories in terms of social mobility and outcomes, ranging from the prospect of death on the street in Brazil to the prospect of stable employment, marriage and children in Nepal (Panter-Brick, 2003).

Programmes limited to increasing knowledge and awareness about HIV and other adverse outcomes of unprotected sex can only expect limited success since the sexual health of young people is inextricably linked to wider social, political and legal contexts. While selling or exchanging sex may be a choice for some, for others, unless other opportunities to diversify their economic activity are available, there may be few or no alternatives. Ironically, campaigns against child labour and legislation that criminalise children's work on the street do little to promote alternatives to the trading or sale of sex as a means of survival (Swift, 1997; Rurevo and Bourdillon, 2003). Similarly, restrictive programmes that remove young people from the street and institutionalise them, or return them to untenable situations from which they have fled, are unlikely to be successful (Rurevo and Bourdillon, 2003). Rather, the programmes more likely to be successful are those that appreciate the problems of children and young people as they experience them themselves, and respect their competence and right to take part in making decisions that affect their lives (Inciardi and Surratt,1997; Rurevo and Bourdillon, 2003; Dybicz, 2005).

In the broader literature of approaches to promoting young people's sexual health, there are examples of how this work can be contextualised. Rather than focusing solely on the sexual health aspects of young people's lives, these needs are addressed through a wider range of activities designed to promote young people's participation in education and other social activities, as well as to support their rights to citizenship, non-discrimination and access to services and support. There are clear similarities between these approaches and the work of the *Streets Ahead* project described earlier.

The *Casa de Passagem* project, in Recife, Brazil (in Barker and Knaul, 2000), for example, offers a drop-in centre for street girls and young women. Food, shelter and medical assistance are provided along with counselling and psychological support. Basic education and vocational training opportunities are also on offer. In addition to these activities, the project runs a preventive health outreach programme. Following an eight month comprehensive training course covering citizens' rights, family planning, body care, sexual abuse, sex education and STI prevention, women's rights, gender and self-esteem, girls and young women become paid health outreach workers for their peers. Activities have included individual and group peer counselling, condom distribution, preventive health-care presentations and health theatre productions.

The *Baaba* project in Kampala, Uganda (International Bank for Reconstruction and Development/The World Bank, 2003) is a peer-led sexual health rights (SHR) project promoting the sexual health of street children. The project works to sensitise all NGOs working with street young people about their sexual health rights and build capacity to meet their sexual and reproductive health needs. A team of 300 'Baabas', or peer educators, provide sexual health and HIV prevention education to other young people on the streets. In addition, 'Baabas' run workshops on the sexual health rights of street children to local councillors, the police and child rights advocates.

The *Street Children Development Centre* in Quezon City in the Philippines (www.geocities.com/sdcincph/), provides an outreach service to street children and young people, focusing on values and life-skills education. These include informal sessions or discussion with children, usually in streets or car parks where children congregate. Topics discussed include self-awareness, sex education, health, HIV and drugs, basic literacy, stress and conflict management, and children's rights and responsibilities. Time is spent by outreach workers in gaining the confidence of street youth. Young people also have access to a health drop-in service. If they develop sexually transmitted infections, these 'windows of vulnerability' are used to encourage young people requiring treatment to enter into health contracts. As part of the contract, young people agree to stay in the health centre for the two week treatment period. This time enables them to get well and provides an opportunity for further health education and prevention work. An important finding from this initiative is that street children have begun to recognise the symptoms of STIs in their clients. They not only reported refusing sexual contact at this point, but also brought clients to the health centre for treatment.

Sexual health promotion interventions, on their own, are unlikely to positively impact on the broader social and economic factors in the lives of street living young people that increase their vulnerability to poor sexual health outcomes. More comprehensive and long-term support for economic, social, environmental and educational welfare is required in order to enable young people living on the street to make positive choices about their sexual health (Ochola, 2000; WERK, 2002; Dybicz, 2005).

This said, however, there are a number of key principles that can be drawn out of the literature and from the case study cited from Zimbabwe which appear to point to a degree of success in enabling services to engage street living young people in sexual health promotion programmes. Services that spend time getting to know young people, and establishing trusting relationships with them, are more likely to have a positive impact on young people's sexual health. Outreach work appears to create a sound basis for understanding the young people's sexual relationships and sexual contexts and for responding appropriately. Most importantly, these services are non-judgemental of young people and their lifestyles and create consistent and caring relationships with young people over time. Such approaches also acknowledge young people's sexuality and promote their rights to sexual health information and services. The above are but a few of many examples of how harnessing the resourcefulness of young people and acknowledging the strength of their own social networks and social capital are vital to the success of programmes designed to promote all aspects of health, including sexual health. Investing time in terms of comprehensive training and support, and remunerating young people for their work as peer educators and leaders, are important components of this approach.

Conclusions

Despite the variability and volatility in the circumstances of young people living on the streets of cities around the world, evidence of resilience and resourcefulness in extreme situations abounds. Sadly, however, relatively little work has been done to understand how young people's capacity to generate their own social capital may be best used to promote their sexual and reproductive health. 'Protecting' the vulnerable from identifiable risks remains the overriding paradigm that informs many responses to children and young people in adverse situations. Applied uncritically, rather than assessing risk and vulnerability as relative to the competences and abilities of young people, such a paradigm ignores the fact that children and young people have varying degrees of agency, resourcefulness and resilience to cope with adversity. An analysis and response that focuses only on de-contextualised and generalised sexual health risks both undermines young people's capacities to analyse and find solutions to their difficulties, and may lead to inappropriate and deficient programmatic responses.

Key principles central to analysis and planning for sexual and reproductive health promotion relevant to young people living on the street therefore fall into five key areas – putting the young person first, promoting meaningful participation, gender equity, a rights based approach, and tackling risk and vulnerability within the distinct context of the young person's life (Aggleton *et al.*, 2004).

Acknowledgements

Thanks go to all staff at the *Streets Ahead* project, Harare, to Catholic Relief Services, Zimbabwe, to Kate Wood who jointly conducted the fieldwork in Zimbabwe and, above all, to all the children and young people in Zimbabwe who shared their experiences with us.

References

Aggleton, P., Chase, E. and Rivers, K. (2004) *HIV/AIDS Prevention and Care among Especially Vulnerable Young People: A framework for action*, Southampton/Geneva: Safe Passages to Adulthood Programme/ World Health Organisation.

Ansell, N. and van Blerk, L. (2004) *HIV/AIDS and Children's Migration in Southern Africa*, Southern African Migration Project, Migration Policy Series No. 33.

Ansell, N. and Young, L. (2004) Enabling households to support successful migration of AIDS orphans in Southern Africa, *AIDS Care*, 16, 3–10.

Aptekar, L. (1991) Are Columbian Children Neglected? The Contribution of Ethnographic and Ethnohistorical Approaches to the Study of Children, *Anthropology and Education Quarterly*, 22, 326–49.

Barker, G. and Knaul, F. (1991) *Exploited Entrepreneurs: Street and working children in developing countries*, New York: CHILDHOPE-USA.

Barker, G. and Knaul, F. with Cassaniga, N. and Schader, A. (2000) *Empowerment in Especially Difficult Circumstances*, London: Intermediate Technology Publications.

Baylies, C. (2002) The impact of AIDS on rural households in Africa: A shock like any other? *Development and Change*, 33, 611–32.

Boyden, J. (2003) *Children Under Fire: Challenging assumptions about children's resilience, children, youth and environments*, 13 (1) (available at: <www.colorado.edu/journals/cye/13_1/Vol13_1Articles/CYE_CurrentIssue_Article_ChildrenUnderFire_Boyden-abstract.htm>).

Chase, E., Wood, K. and Aggleton, P (2006) Is this 'coping'? Survival strategies of orphans and vulnerable children and young people in Zimbabwe, *Journal of Social Development in Africa*, 21, 1, 85–105.

Dybicz, P. (2005) Interventions for street children: An analysis of current best practices, *International Social Work*, 48, 763–71.

De Moura, S. (2005) The prevention of street life among young people in Sao Paulo, Brazil, *International Social Work*, 48(2), 193–200.

Ennew, J. (1994) *Street and Working Children: A guide to planning development*, Manual No.4, London: Save the Children Fund.

Harpham, T. (2003) *Measuring the Social Capital of Children*, Young Lives Working Paper No. 4, London: South Bank University.

Inciardi, J. and Surratt, L.(1997) *Children in the Streets of Brazil: Drug use, crime, violence, and HIV risks* (available at: <www.dreamscanbe.org/view/345>).

International Bank for Reconstruction and Development/World Bank (2003) *Education and HIV/AIDS: A sourcebook of HIV/AIDS prevention programs*, Washington: IBRD/WB (available at: <www.schoolsandhealth.org/Sourcebook/Sec03-08-Ug1.pdf>).

Kudrati, M., Plummer, M., Yousif, N. and others (2002) *Sexual Health and Risk Behaviour of Full-time Street Children in Khartoum, Sudan*, XIVth International AIDS Conference, Abstract No. LbOr04.

Lopi, B. and Kiremire, M.K. (2001) *Invisible Girls: The life circumstances and the legal situation of street girls in Lusaka*, Lusaka: Zambia Association for Research and Development and the Movement of Community Action for the Prevention and Protection of Young People against Poverty, Destitution and Exploitation.

Mann, G. (2004) Separated Children, Care and Support, in J. Boyden and J. de Berry (eds) *Children and Youth on the Frontline: Ethnography, armed conflict and displacement*, Berghahn: Oxford, 3–22.

Marino, R. (2003) *Niños de la Calle*, Montevideo, Uruguay: Ediciones Polifermo.

Morrow, V. (2004) Children's 'social capital': Implications for health and well-being, *Health Education*, 104, 211–25.

Ochola, L. (2000) *Streetchildren and Gangs in African Cities: Guidelines for local authorities*, Urban Management Programme, Working Paper Series 18, Nairobi: Habitat.

Panter-Brick, C. (2003) Street children, human rights and public health: A critique and future directions, *Children and Youth Environments*, 13, 147–71.

Raffaelli, M., Campos, R., Merritt, A., Siquiera, E., Antunes, C., Parker, R., Greco, M., Greco, D. and Halsey, N. (1993) Sexual practices and attitudes of street youth in Belo Horizonte, Brazil, *Social Science and Medicine*, 37(5), 661–70.

Raffaelli, M., Siquiera, E., Payne-Merritt, R., Campos, R., Ude, W., Greco, M., Ruff, A. and Halsey, N. (1995) HIV-related knowledge and risk behaviours of street youth in Belo Hoizonte, Brazil, *AIDS Education and Prevention*, 7, 287–97.

Raffaelli, M., Koller, S., Reppold, C., Kuschick, M., Krum. F. and Bandeira, D. (2000) Gender differences in Brazilian street youth's family circumstances and experiences on the street, *Child Abuse and Neglect*, 24, 1431–41.

Rajani, R. and Kudrati, M. (1996) The varieties of sexual experience of the street children of Mwanza, Tanzania, in S. Zeidenstein and K. Moore (eds) *Learning about Sexuality: A practical beginning,* New York: The Population Council and the International Women's Health Coalition, 301–23.

Rurevo, R. and Bourdillon, M. (2003) *Girls on the Street,* Harare: Weaver Press.

Swart-Kruger, J. and Richter, L. (1997) AIDS-related knowledge, attitudes and behaviour among South African street youth: Reflection on power, sexuality and the autonomous self, *Social Science and Medicine,* 45 (6), 957–66.

Swift, A. (1997) *Children for Social Change: Education for citizenship of street children and working children in Brazil,* Nottingham: Educational Heretics Press.

UNAIDS/UNICEF/USAID (2004) *Children on the Brink: A joint report of new orphan estimates and a framework for action,* New York: UNICEF.

UNICEF (1989) *The United Nations Convention on the Rights of the Child,* New York: UNICEF.

UNICEF (2001) *Orphans and Other Vulnerable Children and Adolescents in Zimbabwe,* New York: UNICEF (available at: <www.unicef.org/evaldatabase/index_14428.html>).

UNICEF (2006) *The State of the World's Children: Excluded and invisible,* New York: UNICEF.

WERK for SNV/GTZ (2002) *The Story of Children Living and Working on the Streets of Nairobi,* Nairobi: Women Educational Researchers of Kenya.

World Health Organisation (2000) *Working with Street children: A training package on substance use, sexual and reproductive health including HIV/AIDS and STDs,* WHO/MSD/MDP/00.14. Geneva: WHO.

Wutoh, A.K., Kumoji, E.K., Wutoh, R.D. and Campusano, G. (2002) *Knowledge and Risk Behaviors of Female Street Children in Ghana,* XIVth International AIDS Conference, Abstract no. E11597.

Chapter 6

Young people's same-sex relationships, sexual health and well-being

Peter Aggleton, Ian Warwick and Paul Boyce

Introduction

Some sixty years ago, the Universal Declaration of Human Rights affirmed that all human beings are equal in dignity, in rights and in freedoms, without distinction of any kind. More recently, there have been growing struggles to delineate and achieve sexual rights or the 'rights of all persons to have control over and decide freely and responsibly on matters related to their sexuality, free of coercion, discrimination and violence' (WHO, 2004: 3).

But what do concepts such as sexuality and sexual rights really mean? Are they useful in advancing agendas in the field of development? And how might these notions be applied to matters of public health in general, and young people's health in particular? These are some of the issues that will be explored in this chapter. The focus is on some of the less-often talked about forms of sexual expression among young people, namely same-sex relationships and practices, and associated sexual identities.

These, we recognise, are topics not often discussed in the international literature. The silence that surrounds them means that the challenge is complex – not least because the terms within which same-sex relationships are often discussed in the West (for example, lesbian/gay/homosexual, bisexual, straight/heterosexual) have limited resonance in many non-Western contexts. Here instead, just as in Europe and North America in the past, such matters, if talked about at all, are often conceived of in respect of local descriptors and vernaculars. And while identities such as 'lesbian' and 'gay' may be ascribed to by some – particularly those with access to travel, television, the Internet and other modern means of communication – more often than not, these same terms are inflected with local meanings.

So, what do we mean by sexuality? Many different definitions can be found in the literature. The World Association for Sexology (1999), for example, sees sexuality as 'an integral part of the personality of every human being [whose] full development depends upon the satisfaction of basic human needs such as desire for contact, intimacy, emotional expression, pleasure, tenderness and love'.

The World Health Organisation's current working definition of sexuality, on the other hand, views sexuality as

> ... a central aspect of being human throughout life [that] encompasses sex, gender identities and roles, sexual orientation, eroticism, pleasure, intimacy and reproduction. Sexuality is experienced and expressed in thoughts, fantasies, desires, beliefs, attitudes, values, behaviours, practices, roles and relationships. [It] is influenced by the interaction of biological, psychological, social, economic, political, cultural, ethical, legal, historical and religious and spiritual factors.
>
> (WHO, 2004: 3)

Fundamentally, sexuality is not so much a 'thing' as a set of sensibilities and social practices that give meaning to life, and which tie to broader social relationships. Ultimately, and in every society, there are many ways of being sexual. There may be dominant forms as well as alternative possibilities. What these different practices are called varies from place to place and from time to time. Some may be understood as the norm; others may be perceived as different.

Sexuality is intrinsically linked to physical acts, yet it is simultaneously conceived in discourse – in words and language. Similar, even identical, acts may have different meanings in different social settings and cultures – sexual in one context, not sexual in another. In interactions between people, interpretations can vary. Some forms of touch, or talk, may be mutually interpreted as expressions of sexuality. Such meanings are not transparent however, since one person's reading of an interaction as sexual may not be shared by the other(s) involved in the communication. Definitions of sexuality are thus dependent on the personal and cultural frames of reference that inform how individuals make sense of their desires.

What then is sexual health? The following definition, developed by the Department of Health in England, places emphasis on equity, diversity and sexual fulfilment alongside the avoidance of negative outcomes.

> Sexual health is an important part of physical and mental health. It is a key part of our identity as human beings together with the fundamental human rights to privacy, a family life and living free from discrimination. Essential elements of good sexual health are equitable relationships and sexual fulfilment with access to information and services to avoid the risk of unintended pregnancy, illness or disease.
>
> (Department of Health, 2001)

And what are sexual rights? Recently, and under the auspices of the World Health Organisation, members of a Technical Consultation on Sexual Health met to consider what these might be. Sexual rights, it was agreed,

'... embrace human rights' and include the right of all persons to, free of coercion, discrimination and violence to: the highest attainable standard of sexual health, and to access to sexual and reproductive health care services; seek, receive and impart information related to sexuality; sexuality education; respect for bodily integrity; choose their partner; decide to be sexually active or not; consensual sexual relations; consensual marriage; decide whether or not, and when, to have children; and pursue a satisfying, safe and pleasurable sexual life.

(WHO, 2004: 3)

Young people and sexuality

As other chapters in this book make clear, the field of young people and sexuality is highly contested. Dominant ideologies and approaches are contradictory in how they would have us understand the issues. On the one hand, it is often claimed that young people should be largely innocent of sexual matters, especially if their energies can be channelled into more wholesome pursuits. On the other hand, Western theories of adolescence see the emergence of adult sexuality and development of a stable sense of self as a key accomplishment of the late teenage years (Erikson, 1968).

The mass media too adopts a somewhat ambivalent stance – with calls for young people's innocence to be 'protected' alongside salacious exposés of school-age sex, teenage pregnancy and young people's involvement in sex work. Nowhere are such contradictions clearer than in the USA where sexually explicit imagery on television, in advertising and on the Internet parallel contemporary demands that young people remain innocent, abstinent and chaste.

To date, much discussion of young people's sexuality has been framed by a somewhat limiting set of assumptions. Central among these are notions of heteronormativity, or the belief that 'adult heterosexuality' is the moral and statistical norm against which all forms of sexual expression should be judged. Also significant though is the belief that adult sexuality is something that one 'grows into', and which thereafter remains relatively fixed. Finally, the dominant assumption is that all the major forms of sexuality and sexual expression are known about and that young people's sexuality must be judged not on its own terms but against these pre-existing patterns and norms.

Sex and gender

Michel Foucault (1976) drew attention to the proliferation of discourses concerning sexuality that came into being in the mid-nineteenth century. At that time, in line with contemporary fascinations with taxonomy, a burgeoning number of sexual types, species and 'perversions' came to be defined. All were assumed to be visible, to the professional eye at least, and all were believed to carry with them particular sensibilities and orientations. For Foucault, sexuality as a system of representational practices is intimately linked to the productive capacity of power, and the capacity to render behaviour both explicable and malleable within particular 'regimes of truth'.

Later writers such as Gayle Rubin (1984) highlighted how gender and sexuality systems intersect and interact. Put quite simply, the one cannot be understood without reference to the other. The heterosexual gender behaviour of many Western men, for example, can only be understood in terms of what it is not – prissy, effeminate and gay. Likewise, dominant patterns of femininity are often defined through their antitheses – being manly, being un-ladylike and being butch. These patterns are true of both rich and poor world contexts, although the sanctions brought to bear for the infringement of local norms may vary.

In the Philippines and in Thailand, *bakla* and *kathoey,* who some have described as 'feminised males' (being biologically male but socially feminine), both celebrate and challenge prevailing gender norms through their adoption of exaggeratedly feminine styles, behaviours and subjectivities – demonstrating in the process something of the malleability of gendered and sexual practices in and across cultures. Throughout Mexico, Central and South America, *travestis* (who are biologically male) may dress and to some extent live as women, adapting their clothing, hair and bodies to the purpose. In Taiwan, T-Po (Tomboy-*femme*) identities have been identified among women involved in same-sex relationships (Chao, 2000). And in countries such as Uganda, Kenya, Namibia, Swaziland and South Africa, same-sex relationships of both traditional (for example, woman–woman marriages and mummy–baby relationships) and modern character (for example, Tommy boy and lesbian identities in all of these countries) have been documented among both young and older women (Morgan and Wieringa, 2005).

Ironically, while such identities are criticised, they are also valued – in the case of men at least. Parts of the fashion industry and numerous beauty parlours and salons are run by *bakla, kathoey* and their counterparts – both young and old – in different countries. The entertainment industry provides opportunities for non-gender normative practices in chat shows, comedy features, serials and *telenovelas.* It is vital to recognise, therefore, that same-sex attracted people (and their stereotypes) are both present and absent in all cultures.

While much is now known about same-sex relationships among adults, rather less is understood about the situation among young people. This relates at least in part to the invisibility of young people's sexuality in general. But it also ties to the illegality of same-sex relationships in some contexts, their moral condemnation and a general lack of concern on the part of those working internationally in the fields of development and public health. Throughout the remainder of this chapter, therefore, we will offer some glimpses into the diversity of identities and practices that exist, as well as their implications for the promotion of young people's sexual and reproductive health.

Diversity and commonality

We will begin by highlighting some of the negative responses there have been to same-sex relations among young people, and the implications of these for sexual health. Our focus here will be on the recent experiences of young gay men in Egypt, *ibbi* and *yoos* in Senegal, and same-sex attracted young women in Thailand. More optimistically, there is growing evidence that same-sex relationships involving young people can be positively responded to, even in contexts where hitherto they were denied. Our focus here will be on recent work among *cacheros* (or young male sex workers) in Costa Rica, young men who have sex with men in India, and same-sex-attracted young women in South Africa.

But before we commence our analysis, a further word of caution. We said earlier that the categories invented by late nineteenth century western science and sexology (homosexual, bisexual and heterosexual) and by the modern day lesbian, gay, bisexual transgender and queer (LGBTQ) movements do scant justice to the diversity of same-sex practices and identities that exist in Western and non-Western contexts. For example, the modern word 'gay' cannot capture the range of modern Western identities and experiences of men who have sex with men. A moment's reflection will reveal that there are many ways of 'being gay' in the West: the experiences of young gay men are markedly different from those who are senior citizens; the young unemployed man in a rural area will lead a different life to the urban professional in his middle years; and the gay churchgoing African-Caribbean man will have responsibilities different to the gay man who has recently become a father with his two lesbian friends.

Moreover, it is not uncommon in many cultures for men to have sex with both women and men – adopting the penetrative role with both – and with their masculinity being confirmed (not questioned) in the process[1]. It is not uncommon too for woman to woman sex to be so shrouded in secrecy such that it is never named or recognised publicly, particularly in strongly gender segregated societies.

Some case study illustrations

Young same-sex attracted men in Egypt

Sex between men has long been documented in North African countries such as Egypt. Ahmad al-Tifashi, who died in Cairo in AD 1253, compiled an extensive collection of homoerotic poems describing sexual relations between men in Egypt, North Africa and across the Arab world (al-Tifashi, 1988). The *mamluk* military elite, which ruled Egypt and Syria from 1249 until 1799, themselves slaves purchased from the steppes of Eurasia, are documented to have practised homosexual relations both among themselves and with young men undergoing military training (Murray, 1997). More recently, a variety of literary genres celebrate sexual relations between men in the modern Egyptian novel (Lagrange, 2000).

Nowadays, as throughout much of North Africa, sex between men in Egypt is a not uncommon practice, although the majority of relationships are conducted with an eye to invisibility, not least because a police crackdown has been in place since the late 1990s, which culminated in over fifty arrests following a police raid on the Queen Boat discotheque in Cairo in May 2001. A Human Rights Watch (2004) report on this incident documents the extensive use of arbitrary arrest, detention, torture and betrayal subsequent to this event. Efforts have also been made to claim that homosexual relations between men constitute an offence to the 'unique norms and evolving practices' of Egypt, despite widespread acknowledgment of the indigenous character of male same-sex relations, and the fact that terms such as *khawalatl* (transvestite dancers) and *kodyana* and *barghal* (denoting those who supposedly adopt the receptive and insertive roles in anal sex) remain in common usage.

In this kind of context – where all men are expected to marry and have children, and where roles between women and men and between many men involved in same-sex relationships are strongly gendered – young same-sex attracted men may find it difficult to cope with the tensions between an historic tradition that celebrated the importance of male same-sex relations, a modern day context in which there are vocal claims for lesbian and gay equality, and a Government that seeks to deny both the past and the present in creating something of a fictitious truth. In this same setting sexual health promotion which recognises the diverse ways in which men may express themselves sexually is conspicuous by its absence, with the result that both men and their male and female partners are put at risk of HIV and other sexually transmitted infections.

Ibbis and yoos in Senegal

In Senegal, the term often used to describe men who have sex with other men – *goor jigen* (man/woman) – describes those men who take the receptive role in sexual relations. The term *faaru gor jigen* (lover of a man/woman) is used to denote the active partner. Similar terms exist in local languages in Burkina Faso, the Gambia and many other West African countries where same-sex attracted men, young and old, are both present and absent in the public domain. Men of female appearance and wearing female clothes have an important role to play in traditional dance troups or *simb* (lion dancers), and in neighbouring Burkina Faso also have an important role to play in baptisms and marriages (Niang *et al.*, 2004).

Among groups of men who have sex with men, the term *ibbi* (to open up) is increasingly used to denote the receptive partner in anal sex, with the term *yoo* describing the one who penetrates. Special relationships may exist between *ibis* and *jeggu-ibbis* or *meru-ibbis* and powerful local women – grandes dames who exert influence at community level. *Ibis* are often involved in the occupations of hair styling, fashion and cosmetics. Crucially, in Senegal as in many other countries same-sex attracted men do not see themselves as having exclusively homosexual behaviour. Recent research has indicated that some 99 per cent report having had sex with a woman at some time and 85 per cent report having had sex with a woman in the last month.

Among the Wolof people of Senegal, male–male sexual relations are seen as *soutara* or 'protected and accepted', yet they are not clearly marked alternatives to heterosexual practices. Dominant social norms mean that such relationships are surrounded by a certain level of respect which forbids others from commenting on them or intervening. That said, *ibis* not infrequently experience a degree of stigmatisation, rejection and violence. They may be rejected by their families, threatened verbally and physically, assaulted and raped. This can render them especially vulnerable to sexually transmitted infections, including HIV. *Yoos,* on the other hand, may not be recognised as such, being indistinguishable from other men. Thus, their particular sexual health circumstances and needs may go unrecognised.

In Senegal, few health care workers are trained or comfortable in treating sexually transmitted infections acquired through male-to-male sex, with the result that self-medication for such infections is especially prevalent. Until recently, there have been few specialised programmes to meet the needs of same-sex attracted men, although things are beginning slowly to change. There are changes too on the identity front, with a few younger men beginning to use the Western term 'gai' to describe themselves, their lifestyles and their behaviour.

Same-sex attracted young women in Thailand

In Thailand, the word *thom* (derived from the English word tomboy) refers to a masculine identified same-sex-attracted woman, while the word *dee* (from the word lady) denotes her counterpart, who appears more stereotypically feminine. Women identifying as *thom* and *dee* can be found living throughout the country, in rural areas as well as in cities. While women's sex relations have been documented throughout Thai history – there are pictorial representations on Budhhist temple murals and court poetry makes reference to sexual activity between women in royal harems – the last few years have seen something of a moral panic about the overt expression of homosexuality, especially between women (Sinnott, 1999). This has found expression in sensationalist news stories concerning Thai young people's adoption of Western styles and fashions of which homosexual behaviour is claimed to be one (Sinnott, 2000).

Yet recent research among young factory working women reveals that *thom–dee* relationships are both widespread and relatively 'ordinary' (Thaweesit, 2004). Significantly, while *thom* may exhibit a masculine persona, dressing in manly ways and effecting male gestures and comportment, *dee* cannot easily be distinguished from other women, being more conventionally feminine in appearance and behaviour. In Muang Mai, where Thaweesit's research took place, *thom* wore male-style haircuts, drove motorcycles of the kind normally bought by men, smoked cigarettes, drank alcohol and eyed up good looking girls. They also took pride in giving pleasure to their girlfriends in sexual relationships. *Dee* on the other hand were more conventionally feminine. Several had had relationships with men, some reporting becoming *dee* after losing faith in men as a result of abandonment, violence and neglect. For a few, the adoption of a *dee* identity offered space to negotiate an alternative way of life apart from patriarchal heterosexual relations.

Significantly, virtually nothing has been written about the sexual health needs of same-sex attracted women in Thailand, with the result that these largely go un-met. Moreover, in keeping with ideologies that deny the presence of same-sex relations between women in Thailand, most if not all sexual and reproductive health programmes in that country persist in assuming that all women are heterosexual and that sexual health risks accrue only through involvement in heterosexual sex. This is far from the truth, there being clear evidence that a wide range of sexually transmitted infections can be transmitted through woman-to-woman sex.

Cacheros in Costa Rica

In Costa Rica, sex between men is legal and sex work is not considered a crime unless it is practiced in a 'scandalous' manner. Both male and female sex workers work in saunas, bars, nightclubs, hotels, on the street and in private homes. While some male sex workers providing services to men may be same-sex attracted, others are involved in heterosexual relationships of different types and durations. Western categories such as 'bisexuality' make little sense of such behaviour, especially in a context (such as Costa Rica) where a culture of *cacherismo* is strong. There is no direct English translation for this term. Its nearest equivalent is that of 'top man'. But this phrase does not capture the complexities of being a man first and foremost, and having sex with both men and women.

In recent work, Schifter has documented elements of *cacherismo* in practice – first in relation to *cacheros* who are the regular lovers of *travestis* (or transgender sex workers) in the red light districts of San Jose, the capital city of Costa Rica (Schifter *et al.*, 1996), second in relation to sex between men in prisons (Schifter *et al.*, *op. cit.*) and, finally, with respect to younger men involved in sex work in a casa (house) of prostitution (Schifter, 1998; Schifter and Aggleton, 1999). In this latter study, the majority of young men interviewed were aged between 15 and 17 and came from lower middle class backgrounds. Most only went to the *casa* at night to find clients and to supplement their incomes. Some were students; others worked in a variety of usually poorly paid occupations. In interview, all distinguished themselves from gays and *locas*, who they believed felt like women or wanted to be women. They, on the other hand, knew themselves to be men. Many had girlfriends and the majority anticipated that they would marry at some point in the future. All indicated that they adopted the penetrative role in oral and anal sex with clients.

Cacheros' counterparts can be found in countries throughout Latin America and in the Spanish speaking Caribbean (see, for example de Moya and Garcia, 1999 and Liguori and Aggleton, 1999). Their existence raises important questions concerning the nature of youthful male sexual desire and its links to dominant forms of masculinity. Importantly, in some countries specialist sexual health programmes have been developed to cater to the needs of such men. In Costa Rica, for example a drop in centre called El Salon, offering education and health services, was established following the work reported on above, and in Mexico, non-governmental organisations carry out HIV/STI prevention education and distribute condoms in bath houses and saunas where *masajistas* (men who provide massage and sexual services) work.

Young same-sex-attracted men in India

Same-sex sexuality in India has arguably become more visible in the wake of HIV and AIDS, and the debates about sexual risk and behaviour that the epidemic has generated. This has helped to bring the needs and circumstances of young same-sex attracted men more into focus, most prominently in the contexts of rights–based activism and health promotion strategies. Nevertheless, same-sex sexuality remains criminalised under Section 377 of the Indian Penal Code, and homophobia has direct and indirect manifestations.

Sexuality activism is finding increased prominence in some university campuses in India. This has been instigated by groups of queer-, gay-, and lesbian identified students, aiming to break silence around experiences of harassment, violence and indirect prejudice experienced by many students. Such activism is helping to create spaces in which young people may be able to develop positive identities based on same-sex sexual orientations (D'Penha and Tarun, 2005).

In other contexts, the experiences and self-understandings of same-sex oriented young men in India are less to do with gay or queer forms of identification. Other, ostensibly more indigenous, forms of non-heterosexual identification have acquired increasing public profile in India over the last decade. One of these is the term *kothi*, a word used by some people in India to articulate non-heterosexual forms of male sexuality, associated with effeminate subjectivities (Reddy, 2005). In the wake of HIV-related interventions, *kothi* has been increasingly consolidated as a term of cultural sexual identity (Cohen, 2005; Boyce, under review). Indeed, a young generation of *kothi* identified men in South Asia have established support groups, Internet fora and rights-based activism that together have helped to establish *kothi* as a contemporary term of sexual identification.

Many young men have sex with other men (both young and old), often in circumstances over which they have little choice. Reports indicate that young men in India commonly have their first sexual experiences at a young age, sometimes with older relatives (Khan, 1996). In some remand homes, for example, sex between boys is reportedly common. However, such actions are not always named as sex acts *per se,* but may be interpreted as a normative aspect of power play between boys and young men, having little or nothing to do with sexual identity (Boyce 2004). The risks in such acts are high, especially as condoms are unlikely to be used in penetrative sex, making HIV transmission a high concern.

Same-sex-attracted women in South Africa

Across Africa, numerous kinds of woman-to-woman sexual relations exist (Morgan and Wieringa, 2005). They include woman-to-woman marriage and the taking of female husbands among the Nuer in the Sudan, the Nandi in Kenya and the Igbo in Nigeria, all of which were documented by missionaries, colonial administrators and anthropologists in the early part of the twentieth century, as well as more recently (Tietmeyer, 1985). They also include sexual-game playing between girls and young women (Kaarsch-Maack, 1911/1975; Bagnol, 1996), mummy–baby relationships (Khumalo and Wieringa, 2005) and other bond friendships. The existence of such relationships, while often not acknowledged and rarely talked about, points to a long indigenous history of erotic relations between women. Overlaid upon these traditional forms and practices, however, are modern variants, some of which tie to western ideas of lesbianism and being gay.

In a recent set of interviews, Kheswa and Wieringa (2005) report on the experiences of a group of same-sex attracted women living in the suburbs of Johannesburg, South Africa. Their accounts reveal many of the difficulties of growing up same-sex attracted in a culture that does not (on an everyday basis at least) recognise and validate sexual relationships between women. Bullying, name-calling and physical and sexual abuse were common in the histories of the young women. As a result, some had felt obliged to enter into sexual relationships with men, most of which were unwanted and many of which were abusive. The responses of the young women's families were on the whole negative and few reported receiving validation or help from relatives when they came out as lesbian.

Such negative responses were in contrast to the support the young women reported receiving within the Johannesburg community of same-sex attracted women and also from the Hope and Unit Metropolitan Community Church which is predominantly attended by gay people locally. Here, they reported feeling valued and accepted, finding opportunities to question received stereotypes of lesbian identities as inevitably *butch* and *femme*, and having the freedom to decide when and how to have children, and how to bring them up. Importantly, the context in which the young women interviewed in this study lived – modern day South Africa – is one in which the rights of same-sex attracted people are guaranteed under the national constitution. Yet it is important to recognise that such guarantees at national level offer little protection on a day to day basis against homophobic relatives and communities that continue to have difficulty responding positively to same-sex attraction and same-sex relationships.

Programmatic implications

In the space available here, we can do little more than point to some of the diversity that exists in young people's sexual experiences and behaviours. Our goal has been not to provide an exhaustive catalogue of all the practices to be found, but to point instead to issues of diversity, highlighting in particular the importance of same-sex relations. We have seen that for many young people (and indeed for many adults) these parallel heterosexual involvements are associated with a range of identities, or what should more accurately be described as 'subject positionings'.

Globally, perhaps only a minority of young people who, either occasionally or regularly, participate in same-sex activities see themselves as lesbian, gay or bisexual. More usually, the practices involved are understood within local terms of reference linked closely to what it is to be a woman or a man. But the picture is made more complex by two things. First, there is the fact that some same-sex practices may never be publicly named, or may be named in ways that make sense to those in the 'know' but which sound like other things to those who are ignorant of them. A good example is offered by the term *maasti*, which in Hindi connotes 'playful mischief', and which is used in India as a euphemism for sex between men as well as for other illicit practices.

Second, there is the impact of globalisation and the spread of modern frames of reference, including the use of terminology and concepts such as lesbian, gay, bisexual, transgender and queer. Increasingly young men and women all over the world are taking up the tropes of gayness – albeit in locally inflected ways – to embrace and engage with the sexual counter-cultures of the West (Altman, 2001).

So what are the implications of this broader picture of sexuality for the promotion of young people's sexual health? If young people are not all the same sexually and if sexual beliefs, practices and identities are context specific, what does this mean for our future work in education, public health and development? These are difficult questions and our answers here can only be provisional. Perhaps the first response we can make is to ensure that future sexual health promotion programmes are built on the identified, rather than assumed, beliefs and practices of young people. It can be all too easy to imagine that we really do know what young people's sexual health beliefs and practices are – or even feel that as adults we can decide what they *should* be.

Of course, it is never possible to put aside completely our assumptions about others. To do so might mean that valuable experiences gained professionally (or personally) are not brought to bear on programmes of sexual health. However, knowledge about the lives and needs of others is always partial and this can be especially so when it comes to issues of sexuality and sexual health, since in the presence of adults young people often feel discouraged to voice what they really think, feel or do.

That said, the challenge of talking about sexuality can apply as much to adults who work with young people as to the young people themselves. Taking the opportunity to make explicit shared and individually held assumptions, values and beliefs is time well spent. Doing this can make it easier to recognise differences and commonalities of perspective among professional colleagues. Even if this proves a difficult exercise to undertake, it can at least highlight some of the challenges that may be encountered when subsequently finding out about young people's experiences and understandings. This, though, raises the importance of recognising and valuing diversity. Without doing so, programmes may at best be irrelevant to young people and can at worst reinforce existing forms of stigma and discrimination.

Sexual diversity can take a number of forms. At the generational level, for example, young people's sexuality-related knowledge, values and practices may vary from those of adults, but may also be continuous with them in certain respects. Furthermore, older young people, such as those in their late teens or early twenties, may understand their relationships, their bodies and their sexualities somewhat differently to 12- to 14-year-olds.

While variations can be identified across communities, groups and individuals, it is important to remain sensitive to the ways that an individual can change over time. For any young person (or adult for that matter), what is felt, thought or done at one point in time or in one place, may be different from that which occurs at another time or place. True enough, for some a same-sex relationship may be a passing phase. Or same-sex behaviours may be influenced by the circumstances of prison or of being at a single-sex boarding school. But then, so too may a young woman's relationship with her boyfriend be for the shorter-term, her real desire resting with a female partner found some years later. A young man's courtship of a young woman may be induced by family pressures – a satisfying sexual relationship with another man not realised until he moves away from his parental home.

Importantly, recognising diversity among young people is not the same as accepting every relationship as it stands. Of concern, here, are coercive, violent or abusive relationships – whether these are among partners of the same or opposite sex. As important as it is to assist young people to pursue a satisfying and pleasurable sexual life, young women and young men have the right not to be coerced into a relationship or to suffer violence within one.

That right co-exists with a more general one. As article 12 of the Convention on the Rights of the Child states, young people are to be involved in decisions that affect them. In recent years, understanding has grown of the many ways in which it is possible to consult, involve and engage young people in the development, implementation and evaluation of programmes. However, what programme planners know they should do and what they actually do can vary considerably. Among other things, adults may be shocked or embarrassed by what they hear. They may break confidentiality and share with others what should remain private. They may use jargon or long words to cover up feelings of inadequacy. They may feel threatened when challenged by those who are younger, or fail to trust young people with money or other project resources.

It is not to be expected that adults automatically possess the skills that promote young people's inclusion and participation in sexual health programmes – but that does not mean these competences cannot be developed. If we are to ensure greater numbers of young people have access to information and resources about sexual health, to avoid the risks associated with unintended pregnancy and sexually transmitted infections and, when they wish, to enjoy sexually fulfilling relationships, we must as professionals decide on our priorities.

As valuable as it is, encountering new ideas about young people's sexuality and sexual relationships will achieve little in itself. However, providing opportunities for dialogue with other professionals and with young people themselves may generate shared understandings that enable us to envisage alternative horizons. To get there will require that we use resources strategically, not to fuel old ways of working but to fire up new professional associations that take to heart the rights of all persons to decide – knowledgeably and responsibly – on matters of love, sexuality and intimacy.

Note

1   See Aggleton (1996) and Aggleton (1999), but also Houlbrook (2005) with respect to the sexual identities and practices of early twentieth-century working-class men in London.

References

Aggleton, P. (1996) *Bisexualities and AIDs: International perspectives*, London: Taylor and Francis.

Aggleton, P. (1999) *Men Who Sell Sex*, London: UCL Press.

Al-Tifashi, A. (1988) *The Delight of Hearts: Or what you will not find in any book*, San Francisco: Gay Sunshine Press.

Altman, D. (2001) *Global Sex*, Chicago: University of Chicago Press.

Bagnol, B. (1996) *Assessment of Sexual orientation in Maputo and Nampula*, unpublished report prepared for the Royal Netherlands Embassy in Maputo.

Boyce, P. (2004) *Men Who Have Sex with Men in Calcutta: Gender, discourse and anthropology*, unpublished PhD thesis, Gender Institute, London School of Economics.

Boyce, P. (under review) Conceiving Kothis: Role, agency and anthropology in the construction of male-to-male sexualities in India, *Medical Anthropology*.

Chao, A. (2000) Global metaphors and local strategies in the construction of Taiwan's lesbian identities, *Culture, Health and Sexuality*, 2(4), 377–90.

Cohen, L. (2005) The Kothi wars: AIDS cosmopolitanism and the morality of classi-fication, in V. Adams and S. Leigh Pigg (eds) *Sex in Development: Science, sexuality and morality in global perspective*, Durham: Duke University Press, 269–303.

de Moya, E.A. and Garcia, R. (1999) Three decades of male sex work in Santo Domingo, in P. Aggleton (ed.) *Men Who Sell Sex*, London: UCL Press, 127–40.

D'Penha, M. and Tarun (2005) Queering the Campus: Lessons from Indian univer-sities, in A. Narrain and G. Bhan (eds) *Because I Have a Voice: Queer politics in India*, New Delhi: Yoda Press, 205–16.

Department of Health (2001) *The National Strategy for Sexual Health and HIV*, London: Department of Health.

Erikson, E. (1968) *Identity, Youth and Crisis*, New York: Norton.

Foucault, M. (1976) *The History of Sexuality, Volume 1*, Harmondsworth: Penguin Books.

Houlbrook, M. (2005) *Queer London – Perils and pleasures in the sexual metropo-lis, 1918–1957*, Chicago: Chicago University Press.

Human Rights Watch (2004) *In a Time of Torture: The assault on justice in Egypt's crackdown on homosexual conduct*, New York: Human Rights Watch.

Kaarsch-Haack, F. (1911, republished 1975) *Das Gleichgesschlechtie Leben der Naturvolker*, New York: Arno Press.

Khan, S. (1996) Under the blanket: Bisexualities and AIDS in India, in P. Aggleton (ed.) *Bisexualities and AIDS – International Perspectives*, London: Taylor and Francis, 161–77.

Kheswa, B. and Wieringa, S. (2005) My attitude in manly ... a girl needs to walk on the aisle: Butch-femme subculture in Johannesburg, South Africa, in R. Morgan and S. Wieringa, (eds) *Tommy Boys, Lesbian Men and Ancestral Wives: Female same-sex practices in Africa*, Johannesburg: Jakana Media, 199–230.

Khumalo, S. and Wieringa, S. (2005) 'I'm the black sheep of my family ...': Same sex sexuality in the corners of Swaziland, in R. Morgan and S. Wieringa (eds) (2005) *Tommy Boys, Lesbian Men and Ancestral Wives: female same-sex practices in Africa*, Johannesburg: Jakana Media, 261–80.

Lagrange, F. (2000) Male homosexuality in modern Arabic literature, in M. Ghoussoub and E. Sinclair-Webb (eds) *Imagined Masculinities: Male identity and culture in the modern Middle East,* London: Saqi Books, 169–98.

Liguori, A-L. and Aggleton, P. (1999) Aspects of male sex work in Mexico City, in P. Aggleton (ed.) *Men who Sell Sex,* London: UCL Press, 103–26.

Morgan, R and Wieringa, S. (eds) (2005) *Tommy Boys, Lesbian Men and Ancestral Wives: Female same-sex practices in Africa,* Johannesburg: Jakana Media.

Murray, S. (1997) Male homosexuality, inheritance rules and the status of women in mediaeval Egypt: The case of the Mamluk, in S. Murray (ed.) *Islamic Homosexualities,* New York: New York University Press, 161–73.

Niang, C., Moreau, A., Bop, C., Compaore, C. and Diagne, M. (2004) *Targeting Vulnerable Groups in National HIV/AIDS Programs – The case of men who have sex with men in Senegal, Burkina Faso and the Gambia,* Africa Region Human Development, Working Papers Series No. 82, Washington DC: World Bank.

Reddy, G. (2005) *With Respect to Sex: Negotiating hijra identity in South India,* Chicago: Chicago University Press.

Rubin, G. (1984) Thinking sex: Notes for a radical theory of the politics of sexuality, in C. Vance (ed.) *Pleasure and Danger: Exploring female sexuality,* New York: Routledge and Kegan Paul, 267–319.

Schifter, J. (1998) *Lila's House: Male prostitution in Latin America,* Binghampton, NY: Harrington Park Press.

Schifter, J. and Aggleton, P. (1999) Cacherismo in a San Jose brothel: Aspects of male sex work in Costa Rica, in P. Aggleton (ed.) *Men who Sell Sex,* London: UCL Press, 141–58.

Schifter, J., Madrigal, J. and Aggleton, P. (1996) Bisexual communities and cultures in Costa Rica, in P. Aggleton (ed.) *Bisexualities and AIDS: International perspectives,* London: Taylor and Francis, 99–120.

Sinnott, M. (1999) Masculinity and tom identity in Thailand, in P. Jackson and G. Sullivan (eds) *Lady Boys, Tom Boys, Rent Boys – Male and female homosexualities in contemporary Thailand,* Binghampton, NY: Harrington Park Press, 97–120.

Sinnott, M. (2000) The semiotics of transgendered sexual identity in the Thai print media: Imagery and discourse of the sexual other, *Culture, Health and Sexuality,* 2(4), 425–40.

Thaweesit, S. (2004) The fluidity of Thai women's gendered and sexual subjectivities, *Culture, Health and Sexuality,* 6(3), 205–20.

Tietmeyer, E. (1985) *Frauen Heiraten Frauen: Studien zur Gynaegamie in Africa,* Hohenschäftlarn: Klaus Renner Verlag.

WHO (2004) *Progress in Reproductive Health Research,* 67, Geneva: World Health Organisation.

World Association for Sexology (1999) *Declaration of Sexual Rights,* adopted August 1999 (available at < www.worldsexology.org/about_sexualrights.asp>).

Chapter 7

Sexual violence and young people's sexual health in developing countries

Intersections

Kate Wood

Introduction

Long the domain of feminist, psychological and criminological research, interest in sexual violence (and more broadly in violence related to gender and sexuality) has widened as a result of the advent of HIV and the subsequent increase in attention to sexuality, gender and human rights. The last decade has seen evidence grow both of the contribution of these kinds of violence to suffering and ill-health worldwide, and their role in influencing sexual (and reproductive) health outcomes, including HIV infection (Maman *et al.*, 2000). Different kinds of violence are interlinked and can be understood from multiple intersecting perspectives, which include individual factors such as psychological history and personal background, socio-cultural norms relating to gender and sexuality, historical processes in particular settings such as conflict and the effects of colonialism, and the workings and exclusions of contemporary local, regional and global political economies.

Due to their often subordinate social position, women – and young women in particular – experience these kinds of violence disproportionately (Gao Rupta, 2002). This explains the widespread use by the World Health Organisation, other United Nations agencies and non-governmental organisations of the term 'gender-based violence', which is broader than 'sexual violence' and refers to multiple kinds of 'physical, sexual or psychological harm or suffering' experienced by girls and women. Women's particular vulnerability as a consequence of widespread gender inequalities has to be recognised; nevertheless, boys and young men also suffer violence relating to their gender and sexuality. Examples include sexual coercion experienced during childhood; physical assault experienced by boys and men who practise non-normative (homosexual or transgendered) sexualities (which tend to be stigmatised, to some degree, in most settings); and sexual violence against boys and men in particular settings, notably while living on the streets or in prison.

This chapter focuses specifically on sexual violence, which according to the World Health Organisation (WHO) (2002a: 149), can be defined as:

Any sexual act, attempt to obtain a sexual act, unwanted sexual comments or advances, or acts to traffic, or otherwise directed, against a person's sexuality using coercion, by any person regardless of their relationship to the victim, in any setting, including but not limited to home and work.

Sexual violence takes numerous forms, and includes rape by strangers and sexual partners; rape by individuals or groups during military conflict; unwanted sexual advances or sexual harassment; sexual abuse of children; forced marriage; denial of the right to use contraception or adopt measures to protect against sexually transmitted infections; forced abortion; violent acts against the sexual integrity of women, including female genital cutting and obligatory virginity inspections; and trafficking of people for the purpose of sexual exploitation (WHO, 2002a).

Multiple approaches have been used to study violence. The health and human rights significance of sexual violence has contributed to a sense of urgency among researchers which has gone some way towards overcoming a historically prevalent fear that writing about sexuality, especially among vulnerable and marginalised individuals, might reinforce stigmatising stereotypes (Vance, 1991; Bourgois, 1995). Violence remains a complex area of research, with important ethical implications (WHO, 2001; Ellsberg *et al.*, 2001); in addition, the inherently contested character of violence creates particular methodological challenges (Robben, 1995). Cultural ways of interpreting and talking about sexual violence may be locally specific and complicated, reflecting dominant gender norms. Anthropological work shows that what may be classified as sexual or violent in some contexts may be seen differently in others (for example, Harvey and Gow, 1994). This underlines the importance of in-depth investigation and of careful contextualisation.

Within public health, epidemiological research mapping risk factors for sexual violence (for example, Koenig *et al.*, 2004) has been conducted in parallel with qualitative approaches that are often short-term and based on individual interviews (for example, Ajuwon *et al.* 2001). Close focus work has contributed more culturally grounded and contextualised perspectives, bringing together culture, history and political economy in explorations of gender and multiple forms of violence ranging from the 'everyday' and interpersonal (for example, Harvey and Gow, 1994) to the collective violence of 'social suffering' in marginalised and resource-poor settings (Farmer, 1992; Kleinman *et al.*, 1997). Multi-disciplinary collaborations (for example, Dobash and Dobash, 1998, Jejeebhoy *et al.*, 2005) and reports produced by non-governmental organisations specialising in human rights and post-conflict work (for example, Human Rights Watch, 1996), are further important sources of knowledge.

Against this backcloth, this chapter considers the most common forms of sexual violence experienced by young people in developing country settings.

The first part outlines the forms and prevalence of common kinds of sexual violence, in particular sexual coercion in childhood, in young people's sexual relationships, in community and institutional settings, and during and after military conflict. The second part considers some of the linkages between violence and sexual health, using three interlinked analytic levels – micro (individual and interpersonal), meso (institutional), and macro (structural).

Forms and prevalence of sexual violence

Sexual coercion in childhood

Sexual coercion in childhood, which is manifested in a continuum of practices and includes various strategies ranging from inducement and threat to explicit violence, remains an emergent area of research in developing country settings, despite its implications for sexual health later in life, and despite the fact that a significant proportion of rape cases brought to the attention of medical and police services in developing countries are children (predominantly girls). In Zimbabwe, for example, the proportion is around half, primarily girls abused by adult men they know, in particular relatives and neighbours (Meursing et al., 1995). Since many cases are settled within and between families, some only come to light once the child has contracted a sexually transmitted infection (STI). In South Africa, nearly a third of the 1.6 per cent of women who reported experiencing sexual abuse before the age of 15 (a likely under-reporting) said that the abuser had been a teacher (Jewkes et al., 2002). Case studies emerging from developing country settings are instructive in revealing that those abusing boys are mostly male and include same-age and older peers, and older men, particularly relatives (Population Council, 2004). Men's experiences of sexual coercion in childhood remain under-researched. In one of the few studies of its kind that has been conducted, six per cent of Nicaraguan men reported having experienced attempted or completed penetration before the age of 13 (Olsson et al., 2000).

Medical, media and popular analyses of the category 'child sexual abuse' have tended to focus on individual psychopathology, failing to provide comprehensive, contextualised explanations for its scale and ubiquity. In particular, these analyses have tended to ignore the intersections between gender relations, cultural notions relating to female and male bodies, locally specific constructions of childhood, and political economy in sustaining and providing space for the sexual abuse of children in particular settings. One contextualising study in Namibia and South Africa (Jewkes et al., 2005), for example, points to multiple cultural factors underpinning sexual coercion of children by adults, including entrenched patriarchal attitudes relating to male sexual entitlement and 'ownership' of female bodies; notions about the sensuality and sexual desirability of teenage girls' bodies;

the supposed 'uncontrollability' of male desire and the blaming of young women for rape through ideas about inappropriate female behaviour; children's historical lack of status; notions of inter-generational 'respect', which can leave children vulnerable to abuse; practices of sexual joking between generations; and the attachment of shame to affected families, leading to secrecy. Relevant contextual phenomena may also include, for example, the fragmentation of extended families in many urban environments, leading to a lack of supervision and under-protection of children; increasing alcohol abuse among men in contexts of high unemployment; and the proliferation of inter-generational sexual relationships (of varying degrees of consensuality), particularly in settings of poverty and where certain material commodities are highly sought-after.

In some regions, sexual coercion is institutionalised and accepted as a normative part of certain kinds of relationship. Non-consensual sex experienced by girls and young women, for example, is often legitimised as part of a range of customary practices, including child marriage (mostly in sub-Saharan Africa and South Asia), wife inheritance in sub-Saharan Africa, and forced marriages of girls to their sexual violators to maintain families' 'honour' in the Middle East (WHO, 2002a). These practices are historically rooted and collectively sanctioned, and are based on culturally specific notions of the body, exchange and consent which fit uncomfortably with the individualism and universalism underlying human rights discourse.

Violence and the politics of gender in young people's sexual relationships

Reflecting a concern with the dynamics of HIV transmission in sexual relationships, the early 1990s saw a proliferation of qualitative studies focusing on condom use, decision-making between sexual partners, and female ability to refuse unsafe sex, particularly among vulnerable groups of women – young women, those living in poverty, drug-users or their partners, African women, and minorities (for example, Schoepf, 1992; Sobo, 1993; McGrath et al., 1993). In conceptualising sexual encounters as located practices variously enacted, negotiated and resisted by individuals in particular situations, this literature shed light on the sometimes violent playing out of power differentials in sexual relationships, and on the impact of this violence on women's sexual safety and autonomy. It further demonstrated that young women's capacity to influence the course of their sexual encounters differs radically between individuals, locations, partnerships and situations. The last decade has seen increasing research attention shift to men and masculinities in developing country settings in relation to sexuality, the dynamics of sexual relationships, and violence (for example, Morrell, 2001; Barker, 2005).

Epidemiological research continues to quantify and map so-called 'intimate partner violence' occurring within sexual relationships, which includes various non-consensual sexual experiences including rape, in addition to physical assault, psychological abuse, a range of controlling behaviours, and femicide (WHO, 2002a, 2002b). Various types of abuse often co-exist in relationships, tend to be repeated over time and are justified through notions of control and discipline (WHO, 2002a, 2002b; Fischbach and Herbert, 1997). While survey data are often not directly comparable due to differences in definitions of abuse, cultural variations in disclosing violence, and some studies not including unmarried women, they are instructive in pointing to the high prevalence of partner violence globally. A review of 48 population-based surveys around the world found that between 10 and 69 per cent of women aged between 15 and 49 reported having been physically assaulted by a male partner at some point in their lives (WHO, 2002a; Garcia-Moreno and Watts, 2000). Surveys conducted with (mostly married) men have also produced high figures of self-reported violent behaviour (Martin, 1999). Physical abuse in pregnancy is common, with, for example, 31 per cent of women reporting it in Egypt, 21 per cent in Saudi Arabia, and 10 per cent in Ethiopia (Campbell, J. et al., 2004). For some young women, abuse can escalate and become life-threatening. The availability of guns in many militarised, post-conflict settings significantly increases women's vulnerability. In some developing countries, certain femicides are disguised within the label of 'customary' practice, such as dowry-related murders in India (Fischbach and Herbert, 1997) and 'honour killings' in Jordan (WHO, 2002a). In one study in eastern Turkey, two thirds of married women thought that they would be killed by their husbands or families if they committed 'adultery' (Ilkkaracan and Women for Women's Human Rights, 1998).

Interest in the dynamics of HIV transmission among the most severely HIV-affected group – young women – has focused attention on particular forms and dynamics of sexual coercion, such as the circumstances of first sex and their relationship to the risk of subsequently experiencing violence and becoming infected with HIV, and the risk factors for experiencing sexual coercion (for example, van der Straten et al., 1998; Coker and Richter, 1998, Koenig et al., 2004). Non-consensual sex involves a continuum of strategies that includes verbal pressure, trickery, threat and rape with a weapon (for example, Wood et al., 1998; Ajuwon et al., 2001). Figures for reported 'forced' first sex range from 14 per cent of Ugandan girls aged between 15 and 19 (Koenig et al., 2004) to 40 per cent in Peru (Caceres et al., 2000). Boys' experiences of sexual coercion by older women, girlfriends and male sexual partners is an emerging research area (for example, Ajuwon et al., 2001; Erulkar, 2004; Marston, 2005).

In many settings, popular understandings of the category of rape are incommensurate with legal definitions, with rape being popularly defined as a sexual violation committed by a man who is not a sexual partner, and with whom therefore there is no prior sexual 'contract' (Jejeebhoy and Bott,

2003). In relation to sexual violence by a sexual partner, the intimate nature of the woman's relationship with the violator, the implicit and assumed sexual 'contract' between them, and the stigma and shame attached to having been raped explains why many young women reconfigure sexual assault by a partner as 'not rape', referring to it by other names. Conversely, the expectation in most settings that unmarried girls maintain 'good' behaviour and an untarnished sexual reputation means that to others (including researchers) some may configure desired sexual experiences as 'forced'. Where sexual partners are older or young women feel indebted to, or induced by them, refusing sex may be difficult (Jejeebhoy and Bott, 2003). Boys may be sexually pressurised through masculinity-related taunting and the weight of social expectation (Marston, 2005).

Anthropological and human rights work in developing countries indicates that women's subordinate social position underpins violence and increases their sexual vulnerability (Gao Rupta, 2002). Broad gender inequalities within patrilineal systems, exemplified by men's rights to land ownership, inheritance and control of resources, are reflected within unequal gender norms and expectations which in turn compromise young women's sexual safety (Maitra and Schensul, 2002). Norms related to young people's sexuality, practices of sexual initiation and sanctioned sexual practice vary across cultural settings, between regions, and between urban and rural populations. However, common features across most settings include the double standard which dictates that female sexuality be intensively controlled and kept under surveillance, while the expectation for men is that sex is a means of achieving adulthood and prestige. Another example is that young women are expected to 'say no' to sex even if they desire it, confusing boundaries of consent. Evidently many young women find non-verbal and indirect ways to express sexual interest and consent (Lambert, 2001); nevertheless, contradictory norms combined with inadequate communication skills complicate young people's negotiation of their sexual lives, and can create space for violence to occur (Asencio, 1999). Young people often lack awareness of their rights. In addition, they often lack support from their families and health professionals in relation to sexual relationships, often because they (girls in particular) are not 'supposed' to be engaged in them (Jejeebhoy and Bott, 2003). Women are often expected to react to violence by displaying culturally desirable traits that reflect local norms of femininity, such as perseverance, acceptance of a woman's 'lot', forgiveness and tolerance.

In many settings, gender hierarchy – the implication that men and women are naturally unequal – is so deeply ingrained as to be 'naturalised' and taken for granted, by many women as well as men. In his ethnographic analysis of gender in Kabyle society in Algeria, Bourdieu (2001) describes this hierarchy, or 'masculine domination', as a form of 'symbolic violence' that is pervasive in the structure of everyday life, often with the unwitting consent of the dominated. Many cultural assumptions follow on from this premise, including the expectation that women should be acquiescent and submissive in the face of male authority, and that decision-making from the beginning of sexual relationships is primarily a male domain. Where girls are married in their early or mid teens, or without their consent, to older men, their vulnerability is reinforced. Violence is frequently used to enforce this expected hierarchy. Male disciplinary rights over women, in particular their female sexual partners and sisters, in situations where young women have behaved in ways considered trangressive, have a long historical trajectory (for example, Mager, 1999). Female infidelity, real or suspected, for example, is known to be the most common trigger for physical violence in young people's sexual relationships. Sexual coercion is often related to issues of sexual access, ownership and control (WHO, 2002a; Wood and Jewkes, 2001).

The questions remain, however, of why some settings are characterised by higher levels of violence than others, and why in a particular setting some men take up violence while others do not, especially given that it may backfire (Barker, 2005). The first question relates to contextual factors, such as the social acceptability of violence as a means of resolving conflict in a particular setting, and a history of military conflict leading to militarisation of a region or country. The second question relates to environmental and psychological factors, including family background, history of abuse, use of alcohol, and level of acceptance of gender-equitable ideas (WHO, 2002a; Barker, 2005).

Multi-disciplinary work on gender (particularly masculinity) and the politics of identity has sought to relate men's use of violence against their sexual partners to a crisis in their sense of manhood. Moore (1994), for example, suggests that an individual's 'fantasies of identity' – in the sense of his notions of how he wants to be, and be seen by others to be – are based on 'fantasies of power and agency in the world', which are closely connected to reputation and social strategies needed to maintain investment in those desired subject-positions. According to this perspective, certain types of behaviour on the part of key others (such as sexual infidelities) provoke a crisis which may have violent repercussions because the female partner's action, whether real or imagined, threatens her partner's self-representations, as well as jeopardising the social evaluations held of him by others, in whose achievement he may have invested great effort. Where an individual's sense of masculinity is under threat, these crises of representation produce feelings of 'thwarting', which may bring the man to use violence against his partner as a strategy of struggle in maintaining his particular invested-in 'fantasies of identity' (Moore, 1994).

The impact of political economy on masculinity is important. Some writers have argued that the relationship between poverty and the perpetration of sexual violence is mediated through forms of crisis in, and reshaping of, masculine identities (for example, Bourgois, 1995; Barker, 2005). This may particularly be the case in deprived contexts where young men find themselves unable to control women or support them economically as their fathers and grandfathers might have done, turning to other strategies to reinforce their sense of masculinity (WHO, 2002a). Young men living in deprived communities with few educational or employment opportunities may also engage in subcultural lifestyles in which certain forms of violence are (in moments) glorified, as a way of resisting hegemonic consensus (Glaser, 1992; Bourgois, 1995; Barker, 2005). Political transition can have a powerful impact on understandings of masculinity. In relation to South Africa, for example, it has been argued that the re-definition of gender and the liberalisation of sexuality entailed by the democratic transition have posed serious challenges to orthodox, mainly authoritarian notions of masculinity, leaving many men with a disempowering sense of irrelevance in the domestic sphere (Morrell, 2001; Walker, 2005).

Other forms of sexual violence in community settings

Common forms of sexual violence occurring in community settings but outside of established sexual partnerships include rape by non-partners, which tends to be more likely to be reported to the police (though remains significantly under-reported) than that occurring within sexual relationships; and group rape. Research on group rape has focused on contexts of profound economic marginalisation, including *line-ups* in urban Papua New Guinea (NSRRT and Jenkins, 1994), teenage group rape as described by crack dealers in Harlem (Bourgois, 1995), *streamlining* and *jackrolling* in South African townships (Mokwena, 1991; Wood, 2005), and *bauk* in Cambodia, often targeting a sex worker or student perceived to be sexually available (Population Council, 2004). In young men's narratives, group rape is linked to certain lifestyles (such as those adopted by street gangs), and to the professed need to put certain young women 'in their place', or punish them for transgressing gender norms – such as engaging in lesbian relationships, being sexually unfaithful to a partner, or refusing one of the group's sexual proposition (for example, Wood, 2005). While group rape is evidently an act of power and masculine bonding, some commentators, notably Bourdieu (2001), have looked further to describe it as motivated by some young men's need to prove their virility to other men. This view suggests that the act is underpinned not necessarily by power, but by fear – of failure to achieve a certain form of masculinity, of exclusion from the group, and of losing respect.

Economic vulnerability can leave girls and young women vulnerable to sexual violence. Young women engaging in sex work face routine violence, including harassment, rape (including by groups of men) and police beatings – especially in settings where sex work is illegal. Violence from customers, locals and police is also reported by boys who sell sex in public spaces in India (Khan, 1999) and on the streets in Brazil (Raffaelli *et al.*, 1993). Sexual violence is often a feature both of economic migration and trafficking, although this remains under-researched (Jejeebhoy and Bott, 2003). Women may be sold into marriage or sexual slavery, particularly by families living in extreme poverty (ILO, 1998). Young women who migrate out of choice for economic reasons may also be forced into sexual relations in return for employment. Their vulnerability is deepened when combined with other disadvantage, such as illegal immigration status.

Sexual violence during and after military conflicts

Rape and sexual torture have long been used as a weapon of war in regions and countries as diverse as Central America, Bangladesh, Algeria, Rwanda, Mozambique, Haiti, Kashmir, Indonesia and Sri Lanka (for example, Human Rights Watch, 1996; Littlewood, 1997; Sideris, 2002). Testimonies of sexual violence in conflict describe incidents of extreme brutality, often occurring on more than one occasion (Physicians for Human Rights, 2002). Significant numbers of girls and women have been affected; it is estimated, for example, that between a quarter and half a million Tutsi women were raped in the Rwandan conflict, many of whom are now known to have been infected with HIV (Human Rights Watch, 1996). Sexual exploitation by militias often continues over time, as in the case of the girls forced to become fighters' 'wives' in northern Uganda, Sierra Leone and other places (Healthlink Worldwide, 2002). Separated or unaccompanied children and girls from single-parent households are especially vulnerable. Boys and young men may also be raped in conflict and during detention. An estimated 4000 Croatian male prisoners were tortured in Serb detention camps, 11 per cent of whom were castrated – some by women (Littlewood, 1997; Oosterhoff *et al.*, 2004).

Rape is often used, whether in an organised or random way, in armed conflicts as a means of reinforcing victims' degradation, subverting community bonds, and as a deliberate tool of 'ethnic cleansing'. Anthropological research on 'mass' wartime rape describes rape in this context as a social rather than individual action, suggesting that group rape is more likely to occur in conflicts in which the state is liminal – as during what Littlewood (1997: 11) calls 'decentred privatised conflicts' such as certain kinds of civil war and counter-insurgency – or in conflicts that feature the partition of a territory and its population, such as Bosnia in 1992–3 and the Punjab in 1947 (Hayden, 2000). Ethnography of the 'work' done by rape in conflict situations and its broader symbolisms in peace-time demonstrates that specific episodes of sexual violence have to be located within other contexts in which harm is committed. Writing about her native Croatia and Bosnia, for instance, Olujuc (1998) considers popular 'body folklore' and local concepts of honour, shame and sexuality as expressed in folk-songs, epic singing, boasting, stories and jokes which construct women's bodies as the symbolic terrain of male competition and microcosm of lineage. Significantly, she argues that war-time rape is a continuation of expressed or enacted violence (symbolic or real) during peace-time.

Sexual violence tends to continue after a military conflict has ended, with refugees and displaced people especially vulnerable to it. In militarised regions, unemployed, traumatised and marginalised young men with continuing access to weapons are likely to become involved in criminal (including sexual) violence. There is some evidence of post-conflict increases in the rape of girls as compared to pre-conflict levels as a result of the 'normalisation' of sexual violence (Save the Children, 2002). For instance, a sharp increase in the number of rapes has been documented for post-invasion Iraq (Human Rights Watch, 2003). In some African countries, national and international peace-keeping forces have been implicated in sexual abuse (Bartolomei *et al.*, 2003). Given the food insecurity, instabilities and displacement of refugee camp life, sex becomes a trading commodity for many girls and young women in these situations. Boys find it easier to enter the marketplace and earn a living (Save the Children, 2002). The abduction and sale of young refugee girls as brides has been documented (Bartolomei *et al.*, 2003). Sexual health is often a lesser priority for humanitarian agencies working with refugees in serious need of material assistance, and sexual violence projects remain limited in number. Other priorities may lead to sexual abuse being ignored, as in the Congolese camps for Rwandan survivors, in which many girls were harassed and raped by armed men whom the international community failed to identify and stop.

A broader view of sexual violence in conflict and post-conflict settings is critical to understanding how multiple forms of human rights violations intersect to produce multi-dimensional vulnerability. Bartolomei *et al.* (2003), for example, analyse why systematic rape happens in one Kenyan refugee camp, considering how the loss and ongoing denial of women's citizenship contributes significantly to their vulnerability. Given the feminisation of poverty in refugee camps, gender discrimination intersects with economic oppression, as well as with discrimination on the basis of ethnic identity. Compounding young women's vulnerability are the loss of state protection suffered by displaced people, the fact that UNHCR guidelines are not enforceable because refugee camps are not sites of citizenship, and their lack of access to health and education services in contexts characterised by the breakdown of basic infrastructure (Save the Children, 2002)

Sexual violence in institutional settings

Sexual violence has been documented, primarily by human rights organisations, in educational institutions, prisons and health-care settings. Schools and tertiary institutions are known to be settings where girls are particularly likely to be sexually harassed or coerced (Mirsky, 2003). One study conducted in South African secondary schools describes girls experiencing a continuum of sexual abuse, including inappropriate touching, unwanted sexual advances, verbal degradation and rape (Human Rights Watch, 2001). Male peers and teachers are both implicated, and usually act with impunity. Sexual relations between teachers and students are not uncommon in many countries, and can begin with a complicated mix of flattery, force and inducement (such as through offers of exam passes). Some girls may reconfigure an incident of coercion as desired after the event.

Sexual expression in prison settings remains an under-researched area in developing countries, but coerced sex and rape are known to be a routine part of establishing hierarchy in prison life. Research has described sexual coercion and the process of becoming a *wyfie* (passive homosexual partner; literally 'wife') in South African prisons (Gear, 2002); the gang rape of unprotected prisoners, those who refuse sexual advances and who change gang allegiance in prisons in Costa Rica (Schifter and Madrigal, 1996); and routine sexual violence, including gang rape, against juvenile prisoners in Malawi (Penal Reform International, 1999). HIV infections are increasing in many prisons, with important public health implications. Reports emerging from South Africa suggest that gang leaders in prisons there are ordering gang members living with HIV to rape disobedient inmates in order to infect them, in a punishment ritual known as 'slow puncture' (Reuters, 2002).

Examples of what WHO classifies as sexual violence in the health sector include obligatory inspections of virginity in Turkey, and forced gynaecological examinations in China (WHO, 2002a).

Connections between violence and sexual health: micro perspectives

While the exact causal pathways between violence and sexual health, including HIV infection, are complex and are not yet fully understood, it is accepted that sexual coercion and violence, combined with the broader gender inequalities underlying them, are significantly linked to multiple forms of sexual (and reproductive) ill-health (Campbell, J., 2002). The links between violence and sexual health, which are both direct and indirect, are known to be four-fold (Maman *et al.*, 2000).

First, physical and sexual violence have direct consequences, increasing young women's vulnerability to STIs (including HIV), sexual difficulties, and negative reproductive health outcomes, including miscarriage, premature labour and low birthweight babies (Caceres *et al.*, 2000; Garcia-Moreno and Watts, 2000; Maman *et al.*, 2000; Dunkle *et al.*, 2004). Forced sex, both vaginal and anal, can increase the risk of HIV transmission through abrasions and injuries, especially in girls, whose vaginal tracts are not fully developed. The biological risk of becoming infected with HIV from rape depends on the type of sexual exposure, the presence of STIs and the degree of trauma. In addition, the theory that violence within sexual relationships plays a role in women's risk of HIV infection was lent support by an important study in urban Tanzania, which found that young HIV-positive women aged 18 to 29 were ten times more likely to report having experienced partner violence than HIV-negative young women (Maman *et al.*, 2001).

Women who have experienced physical and/or sexual violence in relationships are also more likely to report unintended pregnancy and symptoms of reproductive tract infections (Erulkar, 2004). In one South African study, girls who had experienced forced first sex were found to be 14 times more likely to become pregnant in their teenage years (Jewkes *et al.*, 2001). Finally, the connections between partner violence and mental health difficulties, including depression, substance misuse and suicide, have also been documented (Fischbach and Herbert, 1997). The stigma of rape is particularly acute in societies which place great value on pre-marital female virginity. The assumed spoiling of a girl's reputation can bring 'dishonour' on families. In some parts of the world, women who have been raped suffer extreme social ostracism for their perceived defilement (WHO, 2002a). Male rape survivors may feel that their masculinity has been tarnished.

The second, and more indirect, link between violence and sexual health is that the threat of, or actual, violence within sexual partnerships can constrain young women's ability to develop equitable partnerships with men (Wood *et al.*, 1998; Gao Rupta, 2002). In particular, women's reduced autonomy in many inequitable and coercive relationships can impact negatively on their ability to make sexual choices and negotiate the conditions of sexual intercourse, including the use of condoms and contraception. Having a male partner older by five years or more, which is not uncommon in some resource-poor settings, is likely to increase a young woman's vulnerability to HIV in contexts of high prevalence because older men are more likely to be infected with HIV than her male peers. One important mediating dynamic may be that inducement or coercion in these relationships, which are often characterised by resource exchange and sexual obligation, can attenuate young women's agency in influencing the terms of the relationships, including the circumstances of sex.

Third, experiencing sexual coercion during childhood is suspected to increase the likelihood of sexual risk-taking and vulnerability in adulthood, being correlated in young women (mostly in US-based research) with tendencies towards early sexual initiation, alcohol and drug dependence, multiple partners, and unprotected non-contracepting sex (for example, Zierler *et al.*, 1991; Klein and Chao, 1995). This correlation between early sexual abuse and adult risk-taking has been interpreted in psychological terms as connected to poor self-esteem, high personal vulnerability and a tendency to depression, which diminish women's ability and commitment to undertake self-protective practices (Heise *et al.*, 1995). In one study in Nicaragua, women who had experienced attempted or completed rape before the age of 19 were more likely later to have had a higher number of sexual partners compared to non-abused or moderately abused women (Olsson *et al.*, 2000). Qualitative insights into the link between early abuse and risk-taking are emerging from developing country settings. In one study in India, for example, a survivor of childhood incest said that her subsequent relationships with men had become 'sexualised'; another perceived that: 'I was trained as a child to understand my sexuality in ways that made no place for my own wishes and desires. I learned therefore to accommodate the demands of men' (Gupta and Ailawadi, 2004: 3).

The fourth link between violence and sexual health is that for some HIV-positive women, mostly those in sero-discordant relationships, disclosure of their status to their partners brings violence (Garcia-Moreno and Watts, 2000). Fear of violence, rejection and discrimination remains the most commonly cited barrier to disclosure, although a review of available research indicates that it is a minority (between 3.5 and 14.6 per cent) of disclosing women who experience it (Medley *et al.*, 2004).

Violence and sexual health in institutional settings: meso perspectives

Institutions – in particular the health sector, judiciary and law enforcement agencies – have an important role to play in challenging sexual violence. Although important initiatives are taking place to reform institutional responses in some developing countries (WHO, 2002a), in reality the negative effects of sexual violence on individuals and communities are often exacerbated either by an absent, or negative, response to those affected (Jejeebhoy and Bott, 2003). In many settings, health professionals and police respond insensitively to survivors of sexual violence, their responses reflecting wider social norms which – for example – blame young women for their experiences, or construct male prisoners who are raped as 'deserving'. In some environments, authority figures, in particular police, teachers, soldiers and prison warders, are themselves implicated in sexual (and other forms of) violence (Jejeebhoy and Bott, 2003). In most parts of the world, it remains the case that few reported rape cases result in convictions, creating an atmosphere of impunity in which sexual violence is trivialised.

'Structural violence', political economy and sexual health: macro perspectives

In addition to the influence of socio-cultural norms relating to gender identity, individuals' positioning in local, regional and global political economies has a profound influence on their sexual health. Individuals' and communities' vulnerability to experiencing sexual ill-health, including sexual violence, is exacerbated in settings characterised by what some analysts have termed 'structural violence' – a concept developed to describe the myriad forms of social injustices, notably poverty, racism and other inequalities, exclusions and human rights violations which operate at the global, national and local levels (Kleinman *et al.*, 1997; Farmer, 2004). In particular settings, structural factors can make certain groups especially vulnerable, such as migrants, girls and young women, individuals who inject drugs, those from minority groups, people living in profoundly impoverished circumstances, and those dislocated from their communities as a result of conflict.

Sexual ill-health is, for instance, directly linked to conflict (for example, International Crisis Group, 2001); the early rapid spread of HIV in Uganda, for example, has been attributed to the movement, and subsequent demobilisation, of armed forces (Hooper, 1999). Conflict fragments health and education services, renders impossible any national coordinated response to HIV, diverts funding from health, and prevents countries from accessing international financing bodies (Save the Children, 2002). In post-conflict settings characterised by extreme wealth disparities, such as South Africa, Brazil and Guatemala, legacies of violent political struggle, military dictatorship and militarisation form a backdrop to high levels of interpersonal and criminal, including sexual, violence. Structural violence often becomes expressed in everyday, interpersonal violence which in itself brings considerable suffering to communities (Bourgois, 1995, 2001).

While wealth and high status can be linked to sexual ill health, in providing particular kinds of sexual opportunity, sexual health is significantly impacted upon by poverty, marginalisation and processes associated with globalisation and a rapidly changing world economy (Farmer *et al.*, 1996; Baylies, 2000). In many developing countries, it has been argued that structural adjustment programmes, national debt and unfair trade are accentuating poverty and unemployment, which may in turn encourage sexual exploitation (Ghosh *et al.*, 2003). Increasing wealth disparities both regionally and globally open up opportunities for sexual exploitation, visible in high levels of transactional sex, the tourist sex industry operating in many low-income countries, and in the growing commercialisation and commodification of sex (Altman, 2001).

Many developing countries have seen an escalating feminisation of poverty that is linked to sexual ill-health. Economically marginalised women have historically relied on the informal sector, trading commodities to survive. Increasingly, sex is one of those commodities, and sexual clientship networks a means of finding start-up capital (Schoepf, 2002). Young women living in poverty are often forced to engage in activities that jeopardise their sexual health, such as sex work and some forms of transactional sex

(Preston-Whyte *et al.*, 2000). For many girls and women living in settings characterised by resource scarcity and everyday violence, the immediacies of trying to survive make HIV a distant concern (Epele, 2002). For poor families, selling child labour can be a survival strategy, and this can leave children vulnerable to sexual exploitation.

The links between trade, migration and the HIV epidemic are well documented (Haour-Knipe and Rector, 1996). Economic uncertainty has long driven both internal and international migration, particularly in less developed countries. HIV and STI rates are higher in urban areas worldwide, and migration to urban areas – whether permanent, temporary or cyclical – may increase individuals' vulnerability to HIV. Young men who migrate to earn their living through exploitative and often dangerous wage labour, such as in gold mines in South Africa or in logging camps in the Congo, tend to lead lifestyles characterised by the display of fearlessness as a means of coping and in response to the machismo prevailing in these work settings (Campbell, C., 1997; Schoepf, 2002).

Economic and social inequalities occur in every country. Broader violations of rights, or failure to promote rights, have adverse effects on sexual health. Violations of rights such as access to health care and information, food security, and freedom from sexual violence and exploitation may, for example, worsen the impact of HIV, increase vulnerability, and hinder positive responses to the epidemic (Maluwa *et al.*, 2002). Human rights violations are underpinned by existing forms of inequalities and power relations in specific settings, in particular those related to gender, ethnicity, culture and socio-economic status (Parker and Aggleton, 2003). Broad gender-based discrimination, including that relating to marriage, property rights, inheritance, divorce and unequal pay, forms an important background to women's vulnerability to sexual ill-health (Smith-Estelle and Gruskin, 2003). Failure to implement rights frameworks can foster environments in which violence occurs with impunity. Rights violations also have implications for health-seeking; for example, homophobia and the criminalisation of non-normative sexualities in many developing countries makes it difficult for men who have sex with men, or who have been raped, to seek help (Niang *et al.*, 2003; Oosterhoff *et al.*, 2004).

Conclusions

In every society, gender and sexuality are important sites of social, cultural and political contestation. As Amnesty International (2005) articulates, sexual violence is 'rooted in discrimination which denies young women equal rights with men, and which legitimises and sexualises the violent appropriation of women's bodies, whether for individual gratification or political ends'. Both a reflection and cause of human rights violations, sexual violence is compounded by marginalisation and discrimination on the basis of gender, ethnicity, age and socio-economic status. The profound impact of structural violence on young people's sexual health points to the importance of combining macro-level political economic (including historical) explorations with micro-level socio-cultural analysis (Schoepf, 2002; Barker, 2005).

Multi-layered, multi-sectoral approaches are needed for sexual violence prevention and care. Broad programming approaches include individual approaches (such as lifeskills training, programmes for perpetrators and the provision of psychological support), developing health sector responses (including medico-legal services, training for health professionals and comprehensive care for survivors), community-based efforts (such as violence prevention and human rights campaigns and encouraging community activism by men) and school-based programmes, enacting legal and policy responses (including legal reform, and international treaties), and actions to prevent specific forms of sexual violence, such as forced trafficking (see WHO, 2002a). Wider anti-poverty initiatives remain crucial in challenging sexual violence. As many social scientists have pointed out (for example, Parker *et al.*, 2000; Bourdieu, 2001; Schoepf, 2002), the many interventions which are focused on changing consciousness, individual behaviour and group norms are unlikely to succeed on a major scale if they continue to neglect the underlying structural dimensions of sexual ill-health.

References

Ajuwon, A., Oladap Olley, B., Akin-Jimoh, I. and Akintola, O. (2001) Experience of sexual coercion among adolescents in Ibadan, Nigeria, *African Journal of Reproductive Health* 5(3), 120–31.

Altman, D. (2001) *Global Sex,* Chicago: University of Chicago Press.

Amnesty International (2005) *Stop Violence Against Women: Factsheet* (available at: <www.amnestyusa.org/stopviolence/factsheets/sexualviolence.html>).

Asencio, M. (1999) Machos and sluts: Gender, sexuality and violence among a cohort of Puerto Rican adolescents, *Medical Anthropology Quarterly,* 13(1), 107–26.

Barker, G. (2005) *Dying to be Men: Youth, masculinity and social exclusion,* London: Routledge.

Bartolomei, L., Pittaway, E. and Pittaway, E.E. (2003) Who am I? Identity and citizenship in Kakuma refugee camp in northern Kenya, *Development,* 46(3), 87–93.

Baylies, C. (2000) Overview: HIV/AIDS in Africa – Global and local inequalities and responsibilities, *Review of African Political Economy,* 86, 487–500.

Bourdieu, P. (2001) *Masculine Domination* (translated by Richard Nice), Stanford: Stanford University Press.

Bourgois, P. (1995) *In Search of Respect: Selling crack in El Barrio,* New York: Cambridge University Press.

Bourgois, P. (2001) The power of violence in war and peace: Post-Cold War lessons from El Salvador, *Ethnography,* 2(1), 5–34.

Caceres, C., Vanoss, M. and Sid Hudes, E. (2000) Sexual coercion among youth and young adolescents in Lima, Peru, *Journal of Adolescent Health,* 27, 361–7.

Campbell, C. (1997) Migrancy, masculine identities and AIDS: The psychosocial context of HIV transmission on the South African gold mines, *Social Science and Medicine,* 45(2), 273–81.

Campbell, J. (2002) Health consequences of intimate partner violence, *Lancet,* 359, 1131–6.

Campbell, J., Garcia-Moreno, C. and Sharps, P. (2004) Abuse during pregnancy in industrialized and developing countries, *Violence Against Women,* 10(7), 770–89.

Coker, A. and Richter, D. (1998) Violence against women in Sierra Leone: Frequency and correlates of intimate partner violence and forced sexual intercourse, *African Journal of Reproductive Health,* 2(1), 61–72.

Dobash, R. and Dobash, R. (eds) (1998) *Re-thinking Violence Against Women,* London: Sage.

Dunkle, K., Jewkes, R., Brown, H., Yoshihama, M., Gray, G., McIntyre. J. and Harlow, S. (2004) Prevalence and patterns of gender-based violence and revictimization among women attending antenatal clinics in Soweto, South Africa, *American Journal of Epidemiology,* 160, 230–9.

Epele, M. (2002) Gender, violence and HIV: Women's survival in the streets, *Culture, Medicine and Psychiatry,* 26(1), 33–54.

Ellsberg, M., Heise, L., Pena, R., Agurto, S. and Winkvist, A. (2001) Researching domestic violence against women: Methodological and ethical considerations, *Studies in Family Planning,* 32(1), 1–16.

Erulkar, A. (2004) The experience of sexual coercion among young people in Kenya, *International Family Planning Perspectives,* 30(4), 182–9.

Farmer, P. (1992) *AIDS and Accusation: Haiti and the geography of blame,* Berkeley: University of California Press.

Farmer, P. (2004) An anthropology of structural violence, *Current Anthropology,* 45(3), 305–26.

Farmer, P., Connors, M. and Simmons, J. (eds (1996) *Women, Poverty and AIDS: Sex, drugs and structural violence,* Monroe, Maine: Common Courage Press.

Fischbach, R. and Herbert, B. (1997) Domestic violence and mental health: Correlates and conundrums within and across cultures, *Social Science and Medicine,* 45(8), 1161–76.

Gao Rupta, G. (2002) How men's power over women fuels the HIV epidemic, *British Medical Journal,* 324, 183–4.

Garcia-Moreno, C. and Watts, C. (2000) Violence against women: Its importance for HIV/AIDS, *AIDS,* 14 (supp. 3), S253–65.

Gear, S. (2002) *Daii Ding: Sex, sexual violence and coercion in men's prisons,* Research report written for the Centre for the Study of Violence and Reconciliation, South Africa (available at: <www.csvr.org.za/papers/ papsgkn.htm>).

Ghosh, J., Kalipeni, E., Craddock, S. and Oppong, J. (2003) *HIV and AIDS in Africa: Beyond epidemiology,* Oxford: Blackwell.

Glaser, C. (1992) The mark of *Zorro:* Sexuality and gender relations in the *tsotsi* subculture on the Witwatersrand, *African Studies,* 51(1), 47–67.

Gupta, A. and Ailawadi, A. (2004) *Incest in Indian Families: Learnings from a support centre for women survivors,* Presentation at consultative meeting on non-consensual sexual experiences among young people in developing countries,

New Delhi: Population Council, (summary in Population Council (2004) *The Adverse Health and Social Outcomes of Sexual Coercion: Experiences of young women in developing countries* (available at: <www.popcouncil.org/pdfs/popsyn/PopulationSynthesis3.pdf>).

Haour-Knipe, M. and Rector. R. (1996) *Crossing Borders: Migration, ethnicity and AIDS,* London: Taylor and Francis.

Harvey P., and Gow P. (1994) *Sex and Violence: Issues in representation and experience,* London: Routledge.

Hayden, R. (2000) Rape and rape avoidance in ethno-national conflicts: Sexual violence in liminalized states, *American Anthropologist,* 102(1), 36–42.

Healthlink Worldwide (2002) *Combat AIDS: HIV and the World's Armed Forces,* London: Healthlink Worldwide.

Heise, L., Moore, K. and Toubia, N. (1995) *Sexual Coercion and Reproductive Health: A focus on research,* New York: Population Council.

Hooper, E. (1999) *The River: A journey to the source of HIV and AIDS,* London: Penguin.

Human Rights Watch (1996) *Shattered Lives: Sexual violence during the Rwandan genocide and its aftermath* (available at: <www.hrw.org/reports/1996/Rwanda.htm>).

Human Rights Watch (2001) *Scared at School: Sexual violence against girls in South African schools,* New York: Human Rights Watch.

Human Rights Watch (2003) *Climate of Fear: Sexual violence and abduction of women and girls in Baghdad* (available at: <www.hrw.org/reports/2003/iraq0703/2.htm>).

Ilkkaracan, P. and Women for Women's Human Rights (1998) Exploring the context of women's sexuality in Eastern Turkey, *Reproductive Health Matters,* 6(12), 66–75.

International Crisis Group (2001) *HIV/AIDS as a Security Issue in Africa: Lessons from Uganda,* Washington/Brussels: International Crisis Group.

ILO (1998) *The Economics of Sex,* World of Work No. 26, Geneva: International Labour Organisation.

Jejeebhoy, S., Shah, I. and Thapa, S. (2005) *Sex Without Consent: Young people in developing countries,* London: Zed books.

Jejeebhoy, S. and Bott, S. (2003) *Non-consensual Sexual Experiences of Young People: A review of the evidence from developing countries,* New Delhi: Population Council (available at: <www.popcouncil.org/pdfs/wp/seasia/seawp16.pdf>).

Jewkes, R., Vundule, C., Maforah, F. and Jordaan, E. (2001) Relationship dynamics and adolescent pregnancy in South Africa, *Social Science and Medicine,* 52(5), 733–44.

Jewkes, R., Levin, J., Bradshaw, D. and Mbananga, N. (2002) Rape of girls in South Africa, *Lancet,* 359, 319–20.

Jewkes, R., Penn-Kekana, L. and Rose-Junius, H. (2005) 'If they rape me, I can't blame them': Reflections on gender in the social context of child sexual abuse in South Africa and Namibia, *Social Science and Medicine,* 61(8), 1809–20.

Khan, S. (1999) Through a window darkly: Men who sell sex to men in India and Bangladesh, in P. Aggleton (ed.) *Men who Sell Sex: International perspectives on male prostitution and HIV/AIDS,* London: UCL Press, 195–212.

Klein, H. and Chao, B. (1995) Sexual abuse during childhood and adolescence as predictors of HIV-related sexual risk during adulthood among female sexual partners of injection drug users, *Violence against Women*, 1(1), 55–76.

Kleinman, A., Das, V. and Lock, M. (eds) (1997) *Social Suffering*, Berkeley: University of California Press.

Koenig, M., Lutalo, T., Zhao, F., Nalugoda F., Kiwanuka N., Wabwire-Mangen F. (2004) Coercive sex in rural Uganda: Prevalence and associated risk factors, *Social Science and Medicine*, 58, 787–98.

Lambert, H. (2001) Not talking about sex in India: Indirection and the communication of bodily intention, in J. Hendry and C. Watson (eds) *An Anthropology of Indirect Communication*, London: Routledge, 51–67.

Littlewood, R. (1997) Military rape, *Anthropology Today*, 13(2), 7–16.

Mager, A. (1999) *Gender and the Making of a South African Bantustan: A social history of the Ciskei 1945–1959*, Portsmouth: Heinemann.

Maitra, S. and Schensul S. (2002) Reflecting diversity and complexity in marital sexual relationships in a low-income community in Mumbai, *Culture, Health and Sexuality*, 4(2), 133–51.

Maluwa, M., Aggleton, P. and Parker R. (2002) HIV and AIDS-related stigma, discrimination and human rights, *Health and Human Rights*, 6(1), 1–16.

Maman, S., Campbell, J., Sweat, D. and Gielen, A. (2000) The intersections of HIV and violence: Directions for future research and interventions, *Social Science and Medicine*, 50, 459–78.

Maman, S., Mbwambo, J., Hogan, M., Kilonzo G., Sweat M. and Weiss E. (2001) *HIV and Partner Violence: Implications for HIV voluntary counselling and testing programmes in Dar es Salaam, Tanzania*, New York: Horizons, Population Council (available at: <www.popcouncil.org/pdfs/horizons/vctviolence.pdf>).

Marston, C. (2005) What is heterosexual coercion? Interpreting narratives from young people in Mexico City, *Sociology of Health and Illness*, 27(1), 68–91.

Martin, S. (1999) Sexual behaviour and reproductive health outcomes: Associations with wife abuse in India, *Journal of the American Medical Association*, 282, 1967–72.

McGrath, J., Rwabukwali, C., Schumann, D., Pearson-Marks, J., Nakayiwa, S., Namande, B., Nakyobe, L. and Mukasa, R. (1993) Anthropology and AIDS: The cultural context of sexual risk behaviour among urban Baganda women in Kampala, Uganda, *Social Science and Medicine*, 36(4), 429–49.

Medley, A., Garcia-Moreno, C., McGill, S. and Maman S. (2004) Rates, barriers and outcomes of HIV serostatus disclosure among women in developing countries: Implications for prevention of mother-to-child transmission programmes, *World Health Organisation Bulletin*, 82, 299–307.

Meursing, K., Vos, T., Coutinho, O., Moyo, M.,Mpofu, S., Oneko, O., Mundy, V., Dube, S., Mahlangu, M. and Sibindi, F. (1995) Child sexual abuse in Matabeleland, Zimbabwe, *Social Science and Medicine*, 41(12), 1693–1704.

Mirsky, J. (2003) *Beyond Victims and Villains: Addressing sexual violence in the education sector*, Panos Report No. 47, London: Panos Institute.

Mokwena, S. (1991) *The Era of the Jackrollers: Contextualising the rise of youth gangs in Soweto*, Centre for the Study of Violence and Reconciliation, seminar paper no. 7 (available at: <www.csvr.org.za/papers/papmokw.htm>).

Moore, H. (1994) Fantasies of power, and fantasies of identity: Gender, race and violence, in H. Moore (ed.) *A Passion for Difference: Essays in anthropology and gender*, Cambridge: Polity Press, 49–70.

Morrell, R. (ed.) (2001) *Changing Men in Southern Africa*, Pietermaritzburg: University of Natal Press.

Niang, C., Tapsoba, P., Weiss, E., Diagne, M., Niang, Y., Moreau, A., Gomis, D., Wade, A., Seck, K. and Castle, C. (2003) 'It's raining stones': Stigma, violence and HIV vulnerability among men who have sex with men in Dakar, Senegal, *Culture, Health and Sexuality*, 5(6), 499–512.

NSRRT [National Sex and Reproduction Research Team] and Jenkins, C. (1994) *National Study of Sexual and Reproductive Knowledge and Behaviour in Papua New Guinea*, Goroka: Papua New Guinea Institute of Medical Research.

Olsson, A., Ellsberg, M., Berglund, S., Herrera, A,, Zelaya, E., Peña, R., Zelaya, F. and Persson, L.A. (2000) Sexual abuse during childhood and adolescence among Nicaraguan men and women: A population-based survey, *Child Abuse and Neglect*, 24, 1579–89.

Olujic, M. (1998) Embodiment of terror: Gendered violence in peacetime and wartime in Croatia and Bosnia-Herzegovina, *Medical Anthropology Quarterly*, 12(1), 31–50.

Oosterhoff, P., Zwanikken, P. and Ketting, E. (2004) Sexual torture of men in Croatia and other conflict situations: An open secret, *Reproductive Health Matters*, 12(23), 68–77.

Parker, R. and Aggleton, P. (2003) HIV- and AIDS-related stigma and discrimination: A conceptual framework and basis for action, *Social Science and Medicine*, 57, 13–24.

Parker, R., Easton, D. and Klein, C. (2000) Structural barriers and facilitators in HIV prevention: A review of international research, *AIDS*, 14 (Suppl. 1), S22–32.

Penal Reform International (1999) *HIV/AIDS in Malawi Prisons: A study of HIV transmission and the care of prisoners with HIV/AIDS in Zomba, Blantyre and Lilongwe Prisons*, Paris: Penal Reform International.

Physicians for Human Rights (2002) *War-Related Sexual Violence in Sierra Leone: A population-based assessment* ... (Available at: <www.phrusa.org/research/sierra_leone/report.html>).

Population Council (2004) *Sexual Coercion: Young men's experiences as victims and perpetrators*, Research summary (available at: <www.popcouncil.org/pdfs/pop-syn/PopulationSynthesis2.pdf>).

Preston-Whyte, E., Varga, C., Oosthuizen, H., Roberts, R. and Blose, F. (2000) Survival sex and HIV/AIDS in an African city, in R. Parker, R. Barbosa and P. Aggleton (eds) *Framing the Sexual Subject – Studies in gender, sexuality and power*, San Francisco: University of California Press, 165–90.

Raffaelli, M., Campos, R., Merritt, A., Siqueira, E., Antunes, C., Parker, R., Greco, M., Greco, D. and Halsey N. (1993) Sexual practices and attitudes of street youth in Belo Horizonte, Brazil, *Social Science and Medicine*, 37(5), 661–70.

Reuters (2002) *South Africa Prison Gangs use AIDS Rape as Punishment* (available at: <www.aegis.com/news/re/2002/RE021128.html>).

Robben, A. (1995) The politics of truth and emotion among victims and perpetrators of violence, in C. Nordstrom and A. Robben (eds) *Fieldwork Under Fire:*

Contemporary studies of violence and survival, Berkeley: University of California Press, 81–103.

Save the Children (2002) *HIV and Conflict: A double emergency,* London: International Save the Children Alliance.

Schifter, J. and Madrigal, J. (1996) Bisexual communities and cultures in Costa Rica, in P. Aggleton (ed.) *Bisexualities and AIDS: International perspectives,* London: Taylor and Francis, 99–120.

Schoepf, B. (1992) Women at risk: Case-studies from Zaire, in G. Herdt and S. Lindenbaum (eds) *The Time of AIDS: Social analysis, theory and method,* Sage: Newbury Park, 259–87.

Schoepf, B. (2002) 'Mobutu's disease': A social history of AIDS in Kinshasa, *Review of African Political Economy,* 29(93), 561–73.

Sideris, T. (2002) Rape in war and peace: Social context, gender, power and identity, in S. Meintjes, A. Pillay and M. Turshen (eds) *The Aftermath: Women in post-conflict transformation,* New York: Zed Books, 142–58.

Smith-Estelle, A. and Gruskin, S. (2003) Vulnerability to HIV/STIs among rural women from migrant communities in Nepal: A health and human rights framework, *Reproductive Health Matters,* 11(22), 142–51.

Sobo, E. (1993) Inner-city women and AIDS: The benefits of unsafe sex, *Culture, Medicine and Psychiatry,* 17(4), 455–85.

Vance, C. (1991) Anthropology rediscovers sexuality: A theoretical comment, *Social Science and Medicine,* 33(8), 875–84.

Van der Straten, A., King, R., Grinstead, O, Vittinghoff, E., Serufilira, A. and Allen S. (1998) Sexual coercion, physical violence and HIV infection among women in steady relationships in Kigali, Rwanda, *AIDS and Behaviour,* 2(1), 61–73.

Walker, L. (2005) Men behaving differently: South African men since 1994, *Culture, Health and Sexuality,* 7(3), 225–38.

Wood, K. (2005) Contextualising group rape in post-apartheid South Africa, *Culture, Health and Sexuality,* 7(4), 303–17.

Wood, K. and Jewkes, R. (2001) 'Dangerous' love: Reflections on violence among Xhosa township youth, in R. Morrell (ed.) *Changing Men in Southern Africa,* Pietermaritzburg: University of Natal Press, 317–36.

Wood, K., Maforah, F. and Jewkes, R. (1998) 'He forced me to love him': Putting violence on adolescent sexual health agendas, *Social Science and Medicine,* 47(2), 233–42.

WHO (2001) *Putting Women First: Ethical and safety recommendations for research on domestic violence against women,* Geneva: World Health Organisation (available at: <www.who.int/gender/violence/en/womenfirtseng.pdf>).

WHO (2002a) *World Report on Violence and Health,* Geneva: World Health Organisation (available at: <www.who.int/violence_injury_prevention/violence/world_report/en/>).

WHO (2002b) *WHO Multi-country Study on Women's Health and Domestic Violence against Women,* Geneva: World Health Organisation (available at: <www.who.int/gender/violence/en/brochure.pdf>).

Zierler, S., Feingold, L., Laufer, D., Velentgas P., Kantrowitz-Gordon I., Mayer K.. (1991) Adult survivors of childhood sexual abuse and subsequent risk of HIV infection, *American Journal of Public Health,* 81(5), 572–75.

Chapter 8

For love or money

The role of exchange in young people's sexual relationships

Joanna Busza

Introduction

The HIV pandemic has brought the concept of 'transactional sex' to international attention. Although policies and programmes usually target sex work, less formal arrangements where gifts or money are provided within sexual relationships have been found to be widespread and a driving force of the epidemic, particularly in sub-Saharan Africa (Luke, 2003; Côte *et al.*, 2004). Young people appear to be disproportionately involved in economic exchanges for sex, prompting much debate over appropriate responses (Chatterji *et al.*, 2004).

This chapter aims to present the existing evidence concerning young people's participation in sex where exchange plays a significant role, highlight the different forms and meanings of sex for exchange found internationally, and describe and critique various programmes that have been developed so as to meet young people's sexual health needs within the contexts described.

What is sexual exchange?

Simply put, the term 'sexual exchange' indicates the provision of sexual activity in return for payment or other benefits. How such exchanges are negotiated, enacted, and constructed, however, is much more complex. Sex serves as a commodity of exchange along a continuum, from a formalised industry operating within a (usually illegal) market economy, to cultural expectations within emotional relationships that partners should offer gifts or favours. For the purposes of this chapter, however, the following definitions will be used to place sexual exchange into three categories that characterise modern practices and attract increasing attention in the reproductive health field. The majority of empirical evidence from the international health literature describes women trading sex, although both men and women participate in all three forms of sexual exchange.

Sex work is the most easily recognisable from of sexual exchange, consisting of a financial arrangement whereby a client pays a sex worker an agreed fee for sexual services. This can occur in brothels, bars, hotels, saunas, homes, or on the street, and usually represents an occupation or business, in which sex workers engage full-time or on an occasional basis. A distinction is sometimes made between *direct sex work,* which is formalised and takes place in establishments created for the purpose (that is, brothels) and *indirect sex work,* where individuals in certain professions (such as erotic dancers, karaoke singers, bar staff) supplement their income through selling sex on a negotiated basis (Steinfatt, 2002).

Transactional sex refers to the exchange of sex for material support of some kind, including cash, gifts, and economic assistance such as payments for rent or school fees. Although some authors use 'transactional sex' to describe all forms of sexual exchange (Côte *et al.,* 2004), the term generally does not refer to a professional interaction but rather a financial arrangement within other relationships, often characterised by friendship, affection, or romantic attachment.

Survival sex describes the use of sexual exchange as a measure to alleviate extreme poverty or meet immediate economic needs. Survival sex implies that trading sex for money, shelter, food or protection is undertaken out of desperation, literally to ensure survival. This type of exchange is likely to be more sporadic, opportunistic, and unplanned and tends to be reported in situations of instability and deprivation, for instance in refugee camps and among marginalised groups such as drug injectors or street children.

The terms above have been selected for use throughout this chapter due to their relative neutrality. Yet they are all imbued with some controversy, particularly as policy or advocacy efforts attempt to draw delicate moral boundaries across the continuum. For example, the term 'sex work' emerged in the late 1980s and early 1990s as an alternative to 'prostitution' to demonstrate a certain acceptance of sex work as work rather than further stigmatise those involved (NSWP, 1997). Groups that support abolishing sex work prefer the terms 'women in prostitution' or 'victims of prostitution' to highlight sex workers' vulnerability and poor livelihood opportunities (Raymond, 2001). Similarly, numerous alternative terms addressing transactional and survival sex pepper the reproductive health literature, including 'sexual abuse', and 'sexual exploitation', particularly where the participation of young people is involved.

These categories may overlap, and individuals can move between them. Sex workers operating in a brothel or bar environment may subsist on 'pay per act' arrangements, but seek to establish longer-term involvement with greater financial security. A 'client' can become a 'regular' or even a spouse, forming emotional as well as economic attachments (Liao *et al.,* 2003; Agha and Nchima, 2004). Similarly, a transactional arrangement with a 'sugar daddy' or 'mummy' can range from being an established relationship, including bearing children together, to a one-off encounter used to obtain a specific commodity, such as a mobile phone (Longfield *et al.,*

2004). The point at which transactional sex represents someone's sole means of survival also proves difficult to identify, and locally perceived requirements for 'survival' may shift over time.

Finally, terms relating to sexual exchange are likely to invoke different meanings across settings. As many Asian epidemics focused around a brothel-based sex industry, sex work was well recognised by both communities and health authorities, who responded accordingly. On the other hand, they have been slower to react to the growth of informal sexual exchange available in karaoke bars, massage parlours and so on, which often do not meet local definitions of sex work (Hanenberg and Rojanapithayakorn, 1998; VanLandingham and Trujillo, 2002), and much less public health attention appears to have been paid to venues where men may negotiate or sell sex to other men (Storer, 1999). In southern Africa, where sexual networks are more diffuse, the concept of transactional sex may help elucidate how girls' dependence on older men results in their higher infection rates than of their male peers, but does not necessarily mirror indigenous understanding of these behaviours.

While acknowledging weaknesses in attempting to classify a wealth of human experience into three discrete categories, the rest of the chapter will address each in turn, detailing the available evidence of young people's involvement, how this shapes their sexual health, and what programmatic approaches – particularly for HIV prevention – have been adopted in response.

Young people in sex work

Evidence

Reliable data on the extent of young people's participation in sex work are difficult to find. In general, quantifying numbers of sex workers poses great challenges, as sex work is usually illegal and thus hidden. However, many studies suggest that sex workers of both genders tend to be adolescents or young adults. Both quantitative and qualitative studies in developing countries indicate that the majority of sex workers are under the age of 25 (Weir et al., 1998; Larvie, 1999; Baker et al., 2001; Lau et al., 2002). Table 8.1 presents some small-scale surveys conducted with sex worker populations.

The issue of age is sensitive due to internationally agreed United Nations (UN) conventions prohibiting anyone younger than 18 from engaging in sex work. The UN Convention of the Rights of the Child, for instance, obliges governments to protect children from prostitution, while the UN Protocol to Prevent, Suppress and Punish Trafficking in Persons, Especially Women and Children defines all sex workers aged under 18 as having been 'trafficked' regardless of their consent (UN, 2000; Willis and Levy, 2002). In 1999, the International Labour Organization (ILO) categorised sex work as

Table 8.1 Data on age from sex-worker communities

Year of Survey	Population/Location	Findings	Reference
2002	Sex workers in Shenzhen, China, who had been arrested and institutionalised in women's re-education centres	68.5% of 701 under 25 33.3% under 20	(Lau et al., 2002)
2000–2001	Vietnamese brothel-based female sex workers, Phnom Penh, Cambodia	15% of 171 and 10% of 232 women (2 rounds) aged under 18 60% aged 18–20 across both rounds	(Baker et al., 2001)
1996	Female sex workers in diverse venues, Plovdiv, Bulgaria	84% of 200 under 25 26% under 18 4% under 15	(Tchoudomirova et al., 1997)
1995	Qualitative study with 48 female sex workers in a Ugandan trading town	Mean age 25.8	(Pickering et al., 1997)
1992–1998	Brothel-based female sex workers, Bali, Indonesia	4 survey rounds of 620 women Mean age 25.3–26.1	(Ford, K. et al., 2002)
1992–1994	Survey of 172 male sex workers, Casablanca and Marrakech, Morocco	Mean age 24.7	(Boushaba et al., 1999)
1992–1993	Female sex workers in diverse venues, Surabaya, Indonesia	30% of 1,873 aged 25 or younger 29% reported entering sex work aged 10–19 Mean age: 23–29 depending on venue	(Joesoef et al., 2000)
1992	Evaluation of intervention for male sex workers, Rio de Janeiro, Brazil	Majority of 45 participants of qualitative study aged 17–25 (age range 13–38)	(Larvie, 1999)
1990–1991	Female sex workers, Santo Domingo and Puerto Plata, Dominican Republic	Over 50% of 500 under 25	(Weir et al., 1998)

one of 'the worst forms of child labour' (UNICEF, 2000). There is tremendous international pressure to tackle sexual exploitation of children, so where underage sex workers exist, they may lie about their age to avoid legal repercussions, or remain hidden by brothel managers. As a result, there are widely varying estimates of how many children work in the sex industry, with figures up to 10 million quoted, although the methods used to obtain these statistics are rarely described (Willis and Levy, 2002).

The example of Cambodia illustrates the difficulties in establishing an accurate picture of the proportion of sex workers who are underage. In the late 1990s, international hysteria erupted over what was described in the media as 'sex slavery' in Cambodia, with NGOs, politicians, and news reports citing estimates of between 80,000 and 100,000 trafficked female sex workers throughout the country, of whom between 5,000 and 15,000 were alleged to be under the age of 18 years (Bobak, 1996; Steinfatt, 2003). In a rigorous attempt to systematically document the number of sex workers in Cambodia, and estimate the proportion who fitted the UN definition of having been trafficked, Steinfatt (2003) used geographic mapping, census methods, and culturally specific techniques to elicit age. Out of 5,300 directly observed sex workers, Steinfatt determined that just 198 were younger than 18. Box 8.1 presents the experiences of some of Cambodia's young sex workers in their own words.

Implications for sexual health

Younger sex workers are particularly vulnerable to poor sexual health outcomes. For example, among sex workers in Bali, Indonesia, condom use with clients was low (19 per cent), but prevalence of chlamydia or gonorrhoea decreased significantly with age (Ford, K. *et al.*, 2000). This could be due to older women's experience in recognising STI symptoms and seeking treatment, or to a different mix of clients, with those with higher rates of infections patronising younger workers. Furthermore, younger women are biologically more susceptible to HIV (Laga *et al.*, 2001), and unequal power relations vis-à-vis clients and managers will also exacerbate risks. In Thailand, younger women are concentrated in parts of the industry with the poorest conditions, such as low-priced establishments, which attract higher numbers of clients, or those with higher STI rates (Kilmarx *et al.*, 1998).

Younger sex workers can also be at a disadvantage in negotiating condom use. Multivariate analysis of survey results from over 700 sex workers in Shenzhen, China, found that sex workers under the age of 25 were significantly less likely to use condoms and more likely to ever have been diagnosed with an STI than older counterparts (Lau *et al.*, 2002). A survey of Moroccan men selling sex to foreign tourists also found that those aged under 25 were less likely to use condoms (Boushaba *et al.*, 1999). Male sex workers may also be further disadvantaged by prevailing beliefs that anal sex carries fewer risks than vaginal sex, particularly in areas where HIV and AIDS have been portrayed as a disease contracted by men from women (Tan, 1999).

Box 8.1 Brothel based sex work in Cambodia

Thousands of young women from Vietnam have migrated to Cambodia to work in the sex industry. The village of Svay Pak, near the capital Phnom Penh, was well known for its brothels, housing around 300 young sex workers. Most stayed for six months to two years before returning home. Research conducted between 2000 and 2002 elicited sex workers' perceptions, motivations, and concerns. The following interviews are reprinted from Busza (2004).

> My neighbour [told me about Svay Pak] because her daughter was working in Svay Pak ... I saw her daughter making good money to help her family. They were buying a lot of things for their house such as: TV, stereo, fan ...!
>
> (age 18)

> When my mother and I first came, we worked as maids for somebody living in Svay Pak. After two months we didn't save any money and the work was also hard, they looked down on us. I decided to work as a sex worker but my mother disagreed ... But I told her I wanted her to go back to Vietnam and I would work here to earn money, so my mother went home with $100 borrowed from the [brothel] owner ... I also decided to work because I see the sex workers wearing jewelry, it looked like they had an easy life. I have two younger brothers in Vietnam, my father died, so nobody's taking care of us. That's why I decided to work as a sex worker.
>
> (age 16)

> That middleman brought me to Svay Pak ... When she took me to a brothel I knew that they tricked me. I refused to stay in three brothels and I told her I wanted to go home, I didn't want to work here and I was crying. She said if I want to go home, I have to pay her $300 for the transport. I didn't have money ... so I had to stay ...
>
> (age 22)

Programme approaches

Sex work has often been implicated in the spread of HIV, particularly in the early phases of epidemics where they have been classified as 'core transmitters' or a 'reservoir of infection' (D'Costa et al., 1985; NSWP, 1997). A recent study estimates that 84 per cent of HIV prevalence among men in Accra, Ghana, can be attributed to sex work (Côte et al., 2004). Although such findings provoke the blame of sex workers for the spread of a disease, they have also resulted in widespread implementation of HIV prevention programmes that seek to involve sex workers. These can be grouped into three main approaches – control strategies, harm reduction, and empowerment or community mobilisation (Day and Ward, 1997).

Control strategies use the law and criminal justice system to enforce legislative policy. In some cases this involves the arrest and incarceration of sex workers (Lau *et al.*, 2002; Walters, 2004), but often revolves around mandatory STI checks and 'hold orders' that require sex workers to remain in custody for testing and treatment of infections (Potterat *et al.*, 1999). Legal bans on sex work can force the industry underground, potentially increasing risks from violence and reduced access to health services (Ngugi *et al.*, 1999). Other systems seek to regulate conditions in registered establishments. The most famous example of this is the '100 per cent condom policy' initiated in Thailand's brothels, which has been credited with dramatically lowering HIV incidence (Hanenberg *et al.*, 1994) but also criticised for human rights violations (Wolffers and van Beelen, 2003).

'Harm reduction' increases sex workers' access to acceptable sexual and reproductive health services. Clinics that open at convenient hours, peer education, outreach to distribute male and female condoms, lubricant, and referrals to STI treatment comprise some of the strategies employed (Fontanet *et al.*, 1998; Ghys *et al.*, 2001; Ford, K. *et al.*, 2002). While many programmes have increased knowledge and condom use among male and female sex workers, they are not always able to reach communities that do not perceive sexual health as a priority, are constrained by wider structural factors, or marked by hostile and competitive relations rather than supportive networks (Tan, 1999; Campbell, 2000). They also require frequent contact with sex workers and can thus be staff- and resource-intensive.

Empowerment and community mobilisation draw on theories that communities need to address the root causes of powerlessness to bring about sustainable change (Parker, 1996; Beeker *et al.*, 1998). This involves using participatory processes to facilitate the development of critical consciousness, shared identity, and capacity for tackling structural determinants of vulnerability (Chambers, 1994; Kesby, 2000; Paine *et al.*, 2002). Many programmes have adopted this approach (Ford, N.J. and Koetsawang, 1999; Busza and Schunter, 2001; Campbell and McPhail, 2002), with evidence suggesting that those addressing sex workers' concerns beyond health achieve greater success, including in HIV prevention (Evans, 1999; UNAIDS, 2000). In the Sonagachi red light district of Kolkata, India, reported regular condom use with clients rose from 2.7 to 81.7 per cent against a backdrop of political activism, during which sex workers created their own organisation, initiated peer education, and established self-help services (Jana *et al.*, 1998). To what extent the social processes involved in empowerment can be catalysed from outside a community, however, remains unclear (Asthana and Oostvogels, 1996).

Most programmes do not specify particular age groups with which they work. Recently, however, support has increased for 'rescue and rehabilitation' campaigns aimed at sex workers under 18, in order to comply with the UN anti-trafficking convention. The United States Government serves as one of the driving forces behind this approach, which uses raids on brothels or other establishments to liberate underage workers and should include reintegration services such as alternative vocational training, psychosocial support, housing, and health care (Willis and Levy, 2002; Saunders, 2004). There are growing concerns, however, about the way in which such interventions are implemented. Emerging data indicate that organisations that lack understanding of local contexts often undertake 'rescue missions', leading to human rights abuses such as involuntary incarceration (often of adult sex workers), police harassment, and exacerbated socio-economic and physical vulnerability (Jones, 2003; Sutees, 2003; Busza et al., 2004).

Transactional sex

Evidence

Young people's participation in transactional sex is more comprehensively documented due to growing concern that increasing sexual exchange by young people, particularly women, coupled with large age differences between partners, drives the current 'feminisation' of HIV in southern Africa (Laga et al., 2001). As a result, most data come from sub-Saharan Africa, where one analysis of 12 Demographic and Health Surveys (DHS) suggests that between 2 and 27 per cent of women aged 15–19 have engaged in transactional sex (Chatterji et al., 2004). Luke's (2003) comprehensive literature review of quantitative and qualitative studies reporting transactional sex in sub-Saharan Africa found some 45 publications describing women and girls trading sex for favours. These included cash, gifts, make-up, clothes, and school fees elicited from 'sugar daddies' to meet three main objectives – (i) economic assistance, (ii) improved longer-term opportunities, and (iii) increased status among peers (Luke, 2003).

A recent qualitative study from Cameroon found similar motivations for transactional sex, and analysed close to ten different terms used by young people to classify sexual relationships (Longfield, 2004). This study also describes young men seeking sexual relationships for financial gain with older women, known as 'aunties'. Research in Mali has demonstrated that among young people of similar ages, exchange of gifts and money were reciprocated between boys and girls, depending on the strength of the relationship (Castle and Konate, 2003). Data from Asia suggest that while sexual exchange outside a formalised sex industry is less recognised, it does occur. In-depth interviews with young women in Nepal showed that 'adolescent' girls entered sexual relationships in return for money with both older men and male peers (Puri and Busza, 2004). In Cambodian garment factories, young migrant women expect economic support from sexual partners to supplement low incomes (Nishigaya, 2002). Although the sexual health literature tends to overlook examples of men engaging in sex with women for cash and gifts, studies of tourism demonstrate the prevalence of this practice, particularly where local men have opportunities for contact with much wealthier foreigners such as in the Caribbean, Senegal and Gambia, and parts of Central America (Meisch, 1995; Pruitt and LaFont, 1995).

Implications for sexual health

Numerous studies demonstrate associations between transactional sex and low condom use, concurrent and multiple partnerships, and HIV infection (Meekers and Calves, 1997; Kaufman and Stavrou, 2002; Longfield *et al.*, 2004). In a survey of 1395 women attending antenatal services in South Africa, 21.1 per cent reported transactional sex with a non-primary partner, and this group had a 54 per cent increase in the odds of testing HIV positive (Dunkle *et al.*, 2004). Three main pathways lead to this increased vulnerability – dependence on economic benefits, which makes it difficult to risk displeasing (and potentially losing) the partner; symbolic significance of gift-giving, which grants sexual access to the recipient; and the large age differences between young women and their sexual partners that often characterises transactional relationships. Box 8.2 presents a selection of young women's own explanations for engaging in transactional sex, drawn from qualitative research throughout Africa.

Box 8.2 Experiences of transactional sex

Young men and women often express a logical rationale for engaging in transactional sex. The following excerpts from qualitative research conducted in sub-Saharan African countries describe some of their motivations:

> He comes to me to escape frustrations from home ... He takes me out for beer and snacks ... He is my major source of income, and I use him as my *buzi* [goat to milk]
> (19 year-old girl, Tanzania) (Silberschmidt and Rasch, 2001: 1820)

> The main advantage of having many girlfriends is money ... with many girlfriends you increase the chance that one of them can help you when you need it
> (21-year-old male student, Cameroon) (Meekers and Calves, 1997: 368)

> Sugar daddies are better. Why use a pencil when you can use a Bic? ... They are more experienced ... And they don't like to have sex all the time like the young men, and sometimes they have TLC [Tender Loving Care]
> (20 year-old girl, South Africa) (Hunter, 2002: 115)

In many settings, it is the norm for a woman to expect compensation for sex, as a sign of affection or respect (Meekers and Calves, 1997). Kaufman and Stavrou (2002) found that gift-giving carries symbolic meanings in South African young people's sexual negotiation, and different gifts might be reciprocated with different forms of sexual activity. In this study, a girl's acceptance of a gift directly prior to sex, for instance, signified that she had relinquished her right to request a condom. Finally, age 'asymmetries' are statistically associated with decreased condom use and increased HIV prevalence (Gregson *et al.*, 2002), although not all studies have found older men to be most likely to report transactional sex (Chatterji *et al.*, 2004).

Programme approaches

Despite the prominent attention transactional sex now receives, its diversity and widespread cultural acceptance has made it difficult to address. Studies that describe and analyse the practice frequently end with calls for action; for example:

> Enhance adolescent girls' communication skills ... empower them to recognize and prevent unsafe encounters
>
> (Luke, 2003: 77).

> [Provide] information about safer sex practices, including consistent condom use with all types of partners, even those to whom one is emotionally committed ... focus on relationships where young women's risk-taking behaviour is high but risk perception is low.
>
> (Longfield, 2004: 496)

> Encourage these [older] men to adopt safer behaviours. As men still play a dominant role in deciding whether and under what circumstances sex will take place, prevention programmes should focus more on them.
>
> (Laga *et al.*, 2001: 933)

Raising girls' education levels and offering alternative forms of financial support, such as through micro-credit schemes, have also been promoted as 'upstream' intervention approaches (Decosas and Padian, 2002; Kaufman *et al.*, 2004). The extent to which these improve young people's sexual health has not been evaluated, but lack of evidence of a clear association between transactional sex and either socio-economic status or school enrolment suggest that they are unlikely to have large impact (Chatterji *et al.*, 2004).

Unlike in the case of sex work, however, there appears to be greater agreement among researchers that transactional sex, although it may change in form and frequency, retains a traditional role in many societies and thus needs to be absorbed by sexual health promotion approaches, rather than eradicated:

> Certainly, gifts have always been a part of relationships, and this is unlikely to change. The consequences for accepting gifts, however, is likely to have shifted considerably ... [P]rogrammes concerned with safer sex practices should broaden the scope to include gifts as part of the context under which sexual decisions are taken.
>
> (Kaufman and Stavrou, 2002: 389)

Survival sex

The point at which transactional sex becomes 'survival sex' is ambiguous and varies between contexts. Many young people in sex work would argue that their involvement ensures survival and represents a choice only from extremely limited options (Agha and Nchima, 2004; Derks, 2004). Young people in Côte d'Ivoire differentiated a 'prostitute' from someone engaging in transactional sex on the basis of dependence on sexual exchange to meet basic needs such as food and shelter (Longfield, 2004). There is very little information available on young people's involvement in survival sex.

Some examples come from anecdotal reports in conflict and refugee settings, where refugees may trade sex for food, shelter, or protection with other refugees, members of the local host population, or peacekeeping and other military forces (Busza and Lush, 1999; WCRWC, 2001). Internally displaced or migrant communities can also experience levels of instability, marginalisation, and poverty that contribute to reliance on survival sex. An organisation working with street children in Bogota, Columbia, found that many internally displaced 'adolescents' and young people arrived in the city alone, and both girls and boys subsequently sold sex (Ross, 2002). In a situational assessment of migrants throughout Central America, communities reported that border guards demand sex at crossings, while forcibly deported migrants trade sex after having lost their savings (Bronfman *et al.*, 2002). Street children survive through sexual exchange in many settings, and young men who self-identify as homosexual may be forced into dependence on sex work through rejection by parents and communities (Boushaba *et al.*, 1999).

The risks to sexual health are likely to be an exacerbated reflection of those found in transactional sex in general. Studies suggest that the closer to 'survival sex' an exchange becomes, the more likely it is to be marked by low levels of control or negotiating power for the partner receiving economic benefit (Muyinda *et al.*, 2001). Programmes in such settings generally offer basic information, condom distribution, and referrals to health care and subsequently attempt to mitigate the causal vulnerability through poverty alleviation.

Implications for research and policy

If anything, sex for exchange is an area within reproductive and sexual health that has been over-studied. Particularly, once sex work was identified as driving the HIV epidemic in many settings, research expanded significantly, with a focus on developing and evaluating HIV prevention interventions. Controversy followed close behind; sex worker activist groups have increasingly protested against the disproportionate attention they have received as the targets of medical research with few perceived benefits (Singh and Mills, 2005), while changes in the political climate in the USA under the Bush administration led to USAID's removal of financial aid from projects that do not explicitly take an 'anti-prostitution' stand (Saunders, 2004).

Sex for exchange differs in form and meaning across contexts (Harcourt and Donovan, 2005). A full-time brothel-based sex worker in Asia would be unlikely to recognise much in the daily life of a young African woman relying on gifts from her boyfriend or a Latin American man hoping to travel abroad using his romantic contact with wealthy tourists. Some researchers suggest that grouping these phenomena together is thus nonsensical, as local constructs of 'prostitution', 'sugar daddies', 'survival sex', and other terms may not fall along the same continuum, let alone offer direction for the development of programmes (Hunter, 2002). It may not work to apply a 'one-size-fits-all' approach to mitigating sexual health risks of sexual exchange, a criticism levelled at recent US government proclamations as well as rapid scale-up of successful initiatives such as Thailand's '100 per cent condom use' policy (Loff *et al.*, 2003; Busza *et al.*, 2004).

As young people face the challenges and choices in their lives, many will continue to enter sexual relationships involving exchange of money, gifts, or other resources in order to meet immediate or strategic needs. Whether these result in adverse reproductive and sexual health outcomes will depend on the specific mix of social, economic, and political factors shaping each encounter. Is sex consensual? How much scope is there for the negotiation of protection? Do young people have access to the knowledge and services necessary to make responsible decisions in all sexual activity, whether transactional or not? Like other domains of public health, researchers and policy makers need to answer these questions for the contexts in which they work, taking a rights-based approach that encourages young people to define their own realities, needs, and priorities.

Ultimately, while the exchange of money, gifts, or other material support may accompany an imbalance of power in decision making within sexual relationships, the only exchange that actually constitutes a 'risk' for unwanted pregnancy, HIV and other sexually transmitted infections is that of bodily fluids. The concept of 'sexual exchange' may offer a useful framework for analysing certain dynamics behind poor sexual health among young people, but it does not neatly encapsulate one coherent aspect of human sexuality; nor should it distract public health efforts from the basics of sexual health promotion, as Steinfatt (2002) cogently summarised in reference to HIV transmission:

> The virus does not know that the host is a sex worker nor does it seek her out. Nor does the virus know whether the visiting male is a customer, a husband, a lover, or a casual partner ... Sexual transmission of HIV occurs through a specific mechanism: the transmission of bodily fluids, particularly blood and sexual secretions. If these secretions are effectively blocked, as they are through proper use of a condom, the virus is not transmitted.
>
> (Steinfatt, 2002: 234)

References

Agha, S. and Nchima, M.C. (2004) Life-circumstances, working conditions and HIV risk among street and nightclub-based sex workers in Lusaka, Zambia, *Culture, Health and Sexuality,* 6(4), 283–99.

Asthana, S. and Oostvogels, R. (1996) Community participation in HIV prevention: Problems and prospects for community-based strategies among female sex workers in Madras, *Social Science and Medicine,* 43(2), 133–48.

Baker, S., Busza, J., Tienchantuk, P., Ly, S.D., Un, S., Hom, E.X. and Schunter, B.T. (2001) Promotion of community identification and participation in community activities in a population of debt-bonded sex workers in Svay Pak, *6th International Congress on AIDS in Asia and the Pacific, 5–10 October,* Melbourne, Australia.

Beeker, C., Guenther-Grey, C. and Raj, A. (1998) Community empowerment paradigm drift and the primary prevention of HIV/AIDS, *Social Science and Medicine,* 46(7), 831–42.

Bobak, L. (1996) For sale: The innocence of Cambodia, *Ottawa Sun,* Ottawa, 24 October.

Boushaba, A., Tawil, O., Imane, L. and Himmich, H. (1999) Marginalization and vulnerability: Male sex work in Morocco, in P. Aggleton (ed.) *Men who Sell Sex: International perspectives on male prostitution,* London: UCL Press, 263–74.

Bronfman, M.N., Leyva, R., Negroni, M.J. and Rueda, C.M. (2002) Mobile populations and HIV/AIDS in Central America and Mexico: Research for action, *AIDS,* 16 (Suppl 3), S42–S49.

Busza, J. (2004) Sex work and migration: The dangers of oversimplification – a case study of Vietnamese women in Cambodia, *Health and Human Rights,* 7(2), 231–50.

Busza, J. and Lush, L. (1999) Planning reproductive health in conflict: A conceptual framework, *Social Science and Medicine*, 49, 155–71.

Busza, J. and Schunter, B.T. (2001) From competition to community: Participatory learning and action among young, debt-bonded Vietnamese sex workers in Cambodia, *Reproductive Health Matters*, 9, May, 72–81.

Busza, J., Castle, S. and Diarra, A. (2004) Trafficking and health, *British Medical Journal*, 328, 1369–71.

Campbell, C. (2000) Selling sex in the time of aids: The psycho-social context of condom use by sex workers on a southern African mine, *Social Science and Medicine*, 50, 479–94.

Campbell, C. and McPhail, C. (2002) Peer education, gender and the development of critical consciousness: Participatory HIV prevention by South African youth, *Social Science and Medicine*, 55, 331–45.

Castle, S. and Konate, M.K. (2003) Economic transactions associated with sexual intercourse among Malian adolescents: Implications for sexual health, in S. Agyei-Mensah and J.B. Casterline (eds) *Reproduction and Social Context in Sub-Saharan Africa*, Westport: Greenwood Press, 161–86.

Chambers, R. (1994) Participatory rural appraisal (PRA): Challenges, potentials and paradigm, *World Development*, 22(10), 1–17.

Chatterji, M., Murray, N., London, D. and Anglewicz, P. (2004) *The Factors Influencing Transactional Sex among Young Men and Women in 12 Sub-Saharan African Countries*, Washington, DC: Policy Project.

Côte, A.M., Sobela, F., Dzokoto, A., Nzambi, K., Asamoah-Adu, C., Labbe, A.C., Masse, B., Mensah, J., Frost, E. and Pepin, J. (2004) Transactional sex is the driving force in the dynamics of HIV in Accra, Ghana, *AIDS*, 18(6), 917–25.

D'Costa, L.J., Plummer, F., Bowmer, I., Fransen, L., Piot, P., Ronald, A.R. and Nsanze, H. (1985) Prostitutes are a major reservoir or sexually transmitted diseases in Nairobi, Kenya, *Sexually Transmitted Diseases*, 12(2), 64–7.

Day, S. and Ward, H. (1997) Sex workers and the control of sexually transmitted disease, *Genitourinary Medicine*, 73, 161–8.

Decosas, J. and Padian, N. (2002) The profile and context of the epidemics of sexually transmitted infections including HIV in Zimbabwe, *Sexually Transmitted Infections*, 78 (Suppl 1), i40–i46.

Derks, A. (2004) The broken women of Cambodia, in E. Micollier (ed.) *Sexual Cultures in East Asia*, London and New York: Routledge Curzon, 127–55.

Dunkle, K.L., Jewkes, R.K., Brown, H.C., Gray, G.E., McIntyre, J.A. and Harlow, S.D. (2004) Transactional sex among women in Soweto, South Africa: Prevalence, risk factors and association with HIV infection, *Social Science and Medicine*, 59, 1581–92.

Evans, C. (1999) *An International Review of the Rationale, Role and Evaluation of Community Development Approaches in Interventions to Reduce HIV Transmission in Sex Work*, New Delhi: Population Council/Horizons Project.

Fontanet, A.L., Saba, J., Chandelying, V., Sakondhavat, C., Bhiraleus, P., Rugpao, S., Chongsomchai, C., Kiriwat, O., Tovanabutra, S., Dally, L., Lange, J.M. and Rojanapithayakorn, W. (1998) Protection against sexually transmitted diseases by granting sex workers in Thailand the choice of using the male or female condom: Results from a randomized control trial, *AIDS*, 12(14), 1851–59.

Ford, K., Wirawan, D.N., Reed, B.D., Muliawan, P. and Sutarga, M. (2000) AIDS and STD knowledge, condom use and HIV/STD infection among female sex workers in Bali, Indonesia, *AIDS Care,* 12(5), 523–34.

Ford, K., Wirawan, D.N., Reed, B.D., Muliawan, P. and Wolfe, R. (2002) The Bali STD/AIDS study: Evaluation of an intervention for sex workers, *Sexually Transmitted Diseases,* 29(1), 50–8.

Ford, N.J. and Koetsawang, S. (1999) Narrative explorations and self-esteem: Research, intervention and policy of HIV prevention in the sex industry in Thailand, *International Journal of Population Geography,* 5(3), 213–23.

Ghys, P.D., Diallo, M.O., Ettiegne-Traore, V., Satten, G.A., Anoma, C.K., Maurice, C., Kadjo, J.C., Coulibaly, I.M., Wiktor, S.Z., Greenberg, A.E. and Laga, M. (2001) Effect of interventions to control sexually transmitted disease on the incidence of HIV infection in female sex workers, *AIDS,* 15(11), 1421–31.

Gregson, S., Nyamukapa, C., Garnett, G.P., Mason, P.R., Zhuwau, T., Carael, M., Chandiwana, S. and Anderson, R.M. (2002) Sexual mixing patterns and sex-differentials in teenage exposure to HIV infection in rural Zimbabwe, *Lancet,* 359, 1896–903.

Hanenberg, R. and Rojanapithayakorn, W. (1998) Changes in prostitution and the AIDS epidemic in Thailand, *AIDS Care,* 10(1), 69–79.

Hanenberg, R., Rojanapithayakorn, W., Kunasol, P. and Sokal, D. (1994) Impact of Thailand's HIV-control programme as indicated by the decline of sexually transmitted diseases, *Lancet,* 344, 243–5.

Harcourt, C. and Donovan, B. (2005) The many faces of sex work, *Sexually Transmitted Diseases,* 81, 201–6.

Hunter, M. (2002) The materiality of everyday sex: Thinking beyond 'prostitution', *African Studies,* 61(1), 99–120.

Jana, S., Bandyopadhyay, Mukherjee, S., Dutta, N., Basu, I. and Saha, A. (1998) STD/HIV intervention with sex workers, *AIDS,* 12 (Suppl B), S101–S108.

Joesoef, M., Kio, D., Linnan, M., Kamboji, A., Barakbah, Y. and Idajadi, A. (2000) Determinants of condom use in female sex workers in Surabaya, Indonesia, *International Journal of STDs and AIDS,* 11, 262–5.

Jones, M. (2003) Thailand's brothel busters, *Mother Jones,* November/December issue.

Kaufman, C.E. and Stavrou, S.E. (2002) 'Bus fare please': The economics of sex and gifts among young people in urban South Africa, *Culture, Health and Sexuality,* 6(5), 377–91.

Kaufman, C.E., Clark, S., Manzini, N. and May, J. (2004) Communities, opportunities, and adolescents' sexual behaviour in KwaZuluz-Natal, South Africa, *Studies in Family Planning,* 35(4), 261–74.

Kesby, M. (2000) Participatory diagramming as a means to improve communication about sex in rural Zimbabwe: A pilot study, *Social Science and Medicine,* 50, 1723–41.

Kilmarx, P.H., Limpakarnjanarat, K., Mastro, T.D., Saisorn, S., Kaewkungwal, J., Korattana, S., Uthaivoravit, W., Young, N.L., Weniger, B. G. and St. Louis, M.E. (1998) HIV-1 seroconversion in a prospective study of female sex workers in northern Thailand: Continued high incidence among brothel-based women, *AIDS,* 12(14), 1889–98.

Laga, M., Schwartlander, B., Pisani, E., Sow, P. S. and Carael, M. (2001) 'To stem HIV in Africa, prevent transmission to young women', *AIDS*, 15, 7: 931–4.

Larvie, P. (1999) Natural born targets: Male hustlers and AIDS prevention in urban Brazil, in P. Aggleton (ed.) *Men who Sell Sex: International perspectives in male prostitution and AIDS*, London: UCL Press, 159–78.

Lau, J.T.F., Tsui, H.Y., Siah, P.C. and Zhang, K.L. (2002) A study on female sex workers in southern China (Shenzhen): HIV-related knowledge, condom use and STD history, *AIDS Care*, 14(2), 219–33.

Liao, S. S., Schensul, J. and Wolffers, I. (2003) Sex-related health risks and implications for interventions with hospitality women in Hainan, China, *AIDS Education and Prevention*, 15(2), 109–21.

Loff, B., Overs, C. and Longo, P. (2003) Can health programmes lead to mistreatment of sex workers? *Lancet*, 361, 1982–3.

Longfield, K. (2004) Rich fools, spare tyres and boyfriends: Partner categories, relationship dynamics and Ivorian women's risk for STIs and HIV, *Culture, Health and Sexuality*, 6(6), 483–500.

Longfield, K., Glick, A., Waithaka, M. and Berman, J. (2004) Relationships between older men and younger women: Implications for STIs/HIV in Kenya, *Studies in Family Planning*, 35(2), 124–34.

Luke, N. (2003) Age and economic asymmetries in the sexual relationships of adolescent girls in sub-Saharan Africa, *Studies in Family Planning*, 34(2), 67–86.

Meekers, D. and Calves, A.E. (1997) "Main" girlfriends, girlfriends, marriage, and money: The social context of HIV risk behaviour in sub-Saharan Africa, *Health Transition Review*, Supplement to Volume 7, 361–75.

Meisch, L.A. (1995) Gringas and otavelenos: Changing tourist relations, *Annals of Tourism Research*, 22(2), 441–62.

Muyinda, H., Kengeya, J., Pool, R. and Whitworth, J.A.G. (2001) Traditional sex counselling and STI/HIV prevention among young women in rural Uganda, *Culture, Health and Sexuality*, 3(3), 353–61.

Ngugi, E.N., Branigan, E. and Jackson, D.J. (1999) Interventions for commercial sex workers and their clients, in L. Gibney, R.J. Diclemente and S.H. Vermund (eds) *Preventing HIV in Developing Countries: Biomedical and behavioral approaches*, New York: Plenum Press, 205–29.

Nishigaya, K. (2002) Female garment factory workers in Cambodia: Migration, sex work and HIV/AIDS, *Women and Health*, 35(4), 27–42.

NSWP (1997) *Making Sex Work Safe*, London: Network of Sex Work Projects.

Paine, K., Hart, G., Jawo, M., Ceesay, S., Jallow, M., Morison, L., Walvaren, G., Mcadam, K. and Shaw, M. (2002) 'Before we were sleeping, now we are awake': Preliminary evaluation of the Stepping Stones sexual health programme in The Gambia, *African Journal of AIDS Research*, 1, 41–52.

Parker, R.G. (1996) Empowerment, community mobilization and social change in the face of HIV/AIDS, *AIDS*, 10 (Suppl 3), S27–S31.

Pickering, H., Okongo, M., Nnalusiba, B., Bwanika, K. and Whitworth, J.A.G. (1997) Sexual networks in Uganda: Casual and commercial sex in a trading town, *AIDS Care*, 9(2), 199–207.

Potterat, J.J., Rothenberg, R.B., Muth, J.B., Woodhouse, D.E. and Muth, S.Q. (1999) Invoking, monitoring, and relinquishing a public health power, *Sexually Transmitted Diseases*, 26(6), 345–9.

Pruitt, D. and Lafont, S. (1995) For love and money: Romance tourism in Jamaica, *Annals of Tourism Research*, 22(2), 422–40.

Puri, M. and Busza, J. (2004) In forests and factories: Sexual behaviour among young migrant workers in Nepal, *Culture, Health and Sexuality*, 6(2), 145–58.

Raymond, J.G. (2001) *Guide to the New UN Trafficking Protocol*, Amherst: Coalition Against Trafficking in Women.

Ross, T. (2002) Displacement and risk in Colombia, *Research for Sex Work*, 5, 19–20.

Saunders, P. (2004) Prohibiting sex work projects, restricting women's rights: The international impact of the 2003 U.S. Global AIDS Act, *Health and Human Rights*, 7(2), 179–92.

Silberschmidt, M. and Rasch, V. (2001) Adolescent girls, illegal abortions and 'Sugar-daddies' in Dar es Salaam: Vulnerable victims and active social agents, *Social Science and Medicine*, 52, 1815–26.

Singh, J.A. and Mills, E.J. (2005) The abandoned trials of pre-exposure prophylaxis for HIV: What went wrong? *PLoS Medicine*, 2(8), e234.

Steinfatt, T.M. (2002) *Working at the Bar: Sex work and health communication in Thailand*, Westport: Ablex Publishing.

Steinfatt, T.M. (2003) *Measuring the Number of Trafficked Women and Children in Cambodia: A direct observation field study*, Phnom Penh: USAID.

Storer, G. (1999) Bar talk: Thai male sex workers and their customers, in P. Aggleton (ed.) *Men who Sell Sex: International perspectives on male prostitution and AIDS*, London: UCL Press, 223–40.

Sutees, R. (2003) Brothel raids in Indonesia – Ideal solution or further violation? *Research for Sex Work*, 6, 5–7.

Tan, M.L. (1999) Walking the tightrope: Sexual risk and male sex work in the Philippines, in P. Aggleton (ed.) *Men who Sell Sex: International perspectives on male prostitution and AIDS*, London: UCL Press, 241–62.

Tchoudomirova, K., Domeika, M. and Mardh, P-A. (1997) Demographic data on prostitutes from Bulgaria – A recruitment country for international (migratory) prostitutes, *International Journal of STDs and AIDS*, 8, March: 187–91.

UN (2000) *Protocol to Prevent, Suppress and Punish Trafficking in Persons, Especially Women and Children, Supplementing the United National Convention against Transnational Organized Crime*, New York: United Nations.

UNAIDS (2000) *Female Sex Worker HIV Prevention Projects: Lessons learnt from Papua New Guinea, India and Bangladesh*, Geneva: Joint United Nations Programme on HIV/AIDS.

UNICEF East Asia and the Pacific Regional Office (2000) *Children on the Edge: Protecting children from sexual exploitation and trafficking in East Asia and the Pacific*, Bangkok: UNICEF East Asia and the Pacific Regional Office.

VanLandingham, M. and Trujillo, L. (2002) Recent changes in heterosexual attitudes, norms and behaviors among unmarried Thai men: A qualitative analysis, *International Family Planning Perspectives*, 28(1), 6–15.

Walters, I. (2004) Dutiful daughters and temporary wives: Economic dependency on commercial sex in Vietnam, in E. Micollier (ed.) *Sexual Cultures in East Asia*, London and New York: Routledge Curzon, 76–97.

WCRWC (2001) *Refugees and AIDS: What should the humanitarian community do?* New York: Women's Commission for Refugee Women and Children.

Weir, S.S., Fox, L.J., Demoya, A., Gomez, B., Guerrero, E. and Hassig, S.E. (1998) Measuring condom use among sex workers in the Dominican Republic, *International Journal of STDs and AIDS*, 9, 223–6.

Willis, B.M. and Levy, B.S. (2002) Child prostitution: Global health burden, research needs, and interventions, *Lancet*, 359, 1417–22.

Wolffers, I. and Van Beelen, N. (2003) Public health and the human rights of sex workers, *Lancet*, 361, 1981.

Part 3

Chapter 9

Using evaluation to improve the sexual health of young people

Martine Collumbien, Megan Douthwaite and Laboni Jana

Introduction

Funding for health and education programmes is increasingly linked to evidence of effectiveness, defined in terms of measurable health or behavioural outcomes. In part, this is driven by the desire for rapid improvement to reach internationally set targets, such as those agreed at the United Nations General Assembly Special Session (UNGASS) on HIV/AIDS to reduce HIV prevalence among young people (UN, 2001: para 47). Evaluations are sought that can generalise about the key measures to be taken that have potential for large-scale effect, and reviews are required to synthesise the evidence from different studies.

Improving the sexual health of young people, however, requires contextual interventions to effectively target a range of social and environmental influences for enabling and supporting protective behaviour among youth (DiClemente and Wingood, 2003). Because of the inherent context-bound nature of sexual health programmes, there remains debate on how best to produce evidence of effectiveness; what are the successful outcomes to be considered and what are the best designs to measure change in those outcomes?

Evaluation research is, however, not only about evaluating success, but forms an instrumental part of programme design and implementation. It seeks to answer the questions 'what should we do?', 'are we on track?' and, finally, 'did it work, what worked and how?' (Chapman, 2004). Evaluation requires the systematic collection of information to develop local programmes and to study the changes taking place as a result. But evaluation is more than a method of data collection, analysis and interpretation of findings; it offers a way of reasoning. This chapter underlines the potential contribution of evaluation to improving the sexual health of young people in two ways. First, it suggests that programmes can be greatly improved by using findings from evaluation research at all three stages of the programme – design, delivery and results evaluation. Second, it aims to show that the evaluation process and philosophy, and in particular the use of participatory evaluation approaches, can empower both field staff involved in the sexual health work and the young people themelves.

Evaluation for programme improvement: stages throughout the programme cycle

In the health promotion literature, it is conventional to distinguish between process evaluation, which occurs during implementation, and outcome evaluation, which occurs at the end of the intervention. However, evaluation research properly starts at the development stage of a programme with the review of evidence, needs assessment and formative research.

When planning programmes to improve the sexual health of young people, knowledge of 'what works' should inform programme design. This knowledge comes both from theory or other conceptualisations of what should work, and empirical evidence of what *actually* works, derived from other programmes aimed at achieving similar outcomes. Context matters, however. Installing condom machines in women's toilets may 'work' in reducing unprotected sex in societies where girls have both the money and power to negotiate condom use, yet this strategy is bound to be ineffective in contexts where girls are less empowered. Programmes thus need to be designed that are based not only on *general* knowledge about successful intervention approaches, but also on assessments of what is acceptable and appropriate in the *local* context, given the specific needs of the target population.

Formative research provides information for programme design and development. Its findings can sometimes challenge taken-for-granted assumptions. For example, although peer-education is often recommended in community-based programmes, in Kenya formative research has recently revealed that young people preferred to receive information on reproductive health, and referrals to sexual health services, from respected adult counsellors, as this is consistent with local traditions (Erulkar *et al.*, 2004).

Programme activities for or with young people also need to be tested and feedback sought about how they themselves perceived the intervention and what the impact was. Qualitative methods are most often appropriate at this stage, a good example being the use of focus group discussions to pre-test media messages and ensure that they will be well-received and understood (Wellings and Macdowell, 2004).

After programme development, *process evaluation,* often using routine monitoring information, can provide feedback on implementation, and addresses whether the programme is being implemented as planned and is reaching the right young people in the right way. Programmes interact with the environment and rarely go exactly to plan. Process evaluation should therefore be iterative and managers need to course-correct and make improvements if and when needed.

The evaluation of the results of a programme is called *summative* or *outcome evaluation*, and seeks to measure whether the programme achieved its intended effects. Has there been a desired change in health-related behaviour among young people? A pre-specified outcome measure is often used as an indicator of effect – for example, age at first intercourse or reported condom use at last intercourse with a non-regular partner. Since behaviours and attitudes change over time even in the absence of an intervention, observed change needs to be attributable to the programme. This will be discussed in a later section.

In principle, evaluation results should feed back into further planning and improving the local programme. Outcome evaluation results are difficult to interpret without information on context from the process evaluation. It is this combined interpretation and description of results that adds to the existing research evidence of what works.

Not all programmes need an outcome evaluation, and there are several levels of complexity with a wide range of resource implications. Patton (1997) pleads for evaluations to be focused on the primary use of the results – the generation of knowledge (for example, making generalisations about effectiveness and extrapolating principles about what works), judging merit or worth (for accountability often required by donors) and/or improving programmes (identifying weaknesses and strengths for continuous improvement). These three purposes require different evaluation methodologies and may even be in conflict. A primary focus on making generalisations of effectiveness requires the standardisation of programme strategies, which may be incompatible with continuous improvement of the programme. In utilisation-focused evaluation, the main questions to ask in order to focus the evaluation are, who will use the evaluation findings and what decisions will be made on the basis of the evaluation results (Patton, 1997)? These questions help to clarify how complex and precise an evaluation is needed.

Using evaluation to develop effective programmes

Building programme theory

Whatever the purpose of the evaluation, and whoever uses the results, it is crucial to know how the programme or intervention is intended to work before the start. Sexual health programmes operate on the premise that the context (see Chapter 3 in this volume) in which the individual operates has an important bearing on individual behaviour and, therefore, health. Programmes therefore typically combine biomedical, educational and social and policy-orientated elements, and aim to change not only individual health behaviours but also to modify organisations, communities and policies to enable and reinforce this change synergistically.

There is a strong need for improved systematic planning of programmes based on existing research, with much better definition of the objectives and expected outcomes (Nutbeam, 1998). Since even small-scale projects within the field of sexual health promotion can be complex, the biggest contribution of evaluation thinking may well be at the planning and design stage (Coombes, 2004). Patton (1997) has listed a number of principles that need to be thought about at the design stage. These include i) being clear about the goals, purposes and use of the evaluation, ii) being specific about the key variables to be included, iii) focusing and prioritising what can be done and looked at, iv) being systematic in planning and implementing, v) carefully operationalising programme concepts and ideas, and vi) making assumptions explicit by spelling out what can or cannot be done or demonstrated.

So where do we start? What if a certain programme model has been demonstrated to be successful in similar populations and similar contexts? When the aims of the intervention correspond with the community needs, such an approach could be replicated and carefully monitored (assuming that comparable human and financial resources are available). Sometimes the common features of successful programmes in similar populations can guide the design of a new programme (Kirby *et al.*, 1994; McKay, 2000). However, while a review of existing evidence should be an integral part of programme development, the problem definition needs to be based on the epidemiology of the health problem and the needs and goals of the local community. A programme 'theory' can be a helpful starting point in this respect.

A logic model offers a useful tool for developing programme theory. Kirby (2002) has advocated for the use of the behaviour-determinant-intervention (BDI) model as a framework for the development and evaluation of programmes. This model (see Figure 9.1) starts by stating the programme's ultimate health goal. In countries with high HIV prevalence, this goal may focus on reducing transmission of sexually transmitted infections (STIs) and HIV among 15- to 24-year-olds. The next step lies in identifying all the behaviours of young people, groups and institutions that influence the health goal. It is rarely feasible to target all relevant health behaviours, so priorities need to be set according to the local context. For the sake of this example, we focus on increased condom use.

A programme cannot control young people's behaviour directly, but it can change some of its determinants. Thus, the third step is to list all factors plausibly influencing condom use, such as access to condoms, social pressures and opinions of peers, self-esteem, skills in saying 'no' to sex without condoms, perceived personal risk and so on. Based on theory, evidence and feasibility, determinants with the greatest likely impact are then chosen. The final step to complete the model is to explore and select intervention components and activities designed specifically to change each selected determinant.

Building the model from the direction of the health goal to the programme activities (see the top row of Figure 9.1), provides a clear rationale for the structure of the intervention and can act as a guide to programme staff. It makes theoretical assumptions explicit. For evaluation purposes, it is read in the other direction – this is discussed later.

To illustrate this process further, we will use the example of condom social marketing to young people, a practice which is both highly theory-driven and research based. Social marketers focus on those determinants of condom use that are theoretically amenable to change by social marketing intervention strategies. They frequently distinguish between opportunity, ability and motivation factors (Rothschild, 1999; Chapman, 2004). *Opportunity* factors, such as availability and brand appeal, are defined as service-related factors that influence the individual's use of condoms, yet which are beyond his/her control. Affordability, social norms and support, and self-efficacy all influence the *ability* of a young person to act, given the opportunity and the motivation. A person's *motivation* is influenced by the expected benefit of using a condom and their perceived personal risk based on awareness of the health problem, its severity and its causes.

To find out which factors are most important in a particular local setting, data are collected among the target group. First, qualitative research may be used to operationalise the different opportunity, ability and motivation constructs into a set of questions relevant to the local culture (Chapman, 2004). Research conducted among young people in Tanzania, for example, found that trust was often cited as a reason for not using condoms consistently with a primary partner. The research also found that caution and assurance

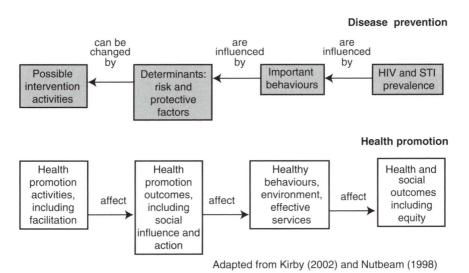

Adapted from Kirby (2002) and Nutbeam (1998)

Figure 9.1 Building and using a logic model

were key elements of trust. Those who were more cautious were less likely to cite trust as a reason for non-use than were those who were less cautious. As might be expected, levels of trust tended to be highest among young married couples, despite the fact that the majority of HIV infections occur within marriage (Klein and Coombes, 2005).

Secondly, a quantitative survey may be conducted to collect information on each potential determinant, and an analysis conducted to compare condom users with non-users to identify significant differences between them in terms of those determinants. To maximise the likelihood that non-users will start using condoms, campaign messages and strategies should focus on influencing the most significant determinants. In Tanzania, specific recommendations were made to target young married couples regarding levels of caution, without reducing overall levels of trust within marriage (Klein and Coombes, 2005). The change in indicators for the reduced set of determinants can then be monitored for progress and evaluated for success.

In this particular example, theoretical constructs were drawn from a range of individual psychosocial models of behaviour change, social learning theory, diffusion of innovation and marketing theory (Chapman, 2004). While most behaviour change theories originated in the richer countries, by selecting relevant constructs and adapting them to poorer countries' local cultures, programmes can be made more effective (Fishbein, 2000). Of particular importance within developing-world contexts are community norms and traditional practices, which strongly influence behaviour. There is a need to aim at bringing about changes at the community level to make behaviours like condom use acceptable (Odutolu, 2005).

Improving sexual health is not simply about disease prevention through individual behaviour change and improved service delivery. Sexual and reproductive health interventions for young people typically aim to i) create a supportive environment for young people, ii) improve their sexual and reproductive knowledge, attitudes, skills and behaviours, and iii) increase utilisation of health and related services (Speizer *et al.*, 2003). The shift of emphasis from a disease prevention to a health promotion framework is represented by contrasting the top and bottom rows of boxes in Figure 9.1. In Nutbeam's (1998) outcome model for health promotion, healthy lifestyles (behaviour), effective health services and healthy environments are all needed to achieve the ultimate goal of positive health and social outcomes, including equity. From a health promotion perspective, encouraging young people to adopt and maintain healthy lifestyles and behaviours is crucial, and requires that young people, parents, communities, local organisations, and other such stakeholders become active participants in shaping healthy lifestyles and policies (Potvin *et al.*, 2001).

Involving young people and the community in the planning process

Young people can and should be readily involved in the development of programmatic approaches using participatory learning strategies (Kirby, 2002). Other community stakeholders, programme staff and people knowledgeable about the research evidence can all form part of a working group to help develop the model. Ensuring that young people's voices are heard may mean gaining their input in separate meetings, or simply engaging with them in the community during this planning stage.

A successful example of involving young people and the community in the planning process is provided by the Child In Need Institute (CINI), a large NGO in India, implementing a Young People's Reproductive and Sexual Health Programme in a peri-urban community near Kolkata. Since the work was funded as a demonstration project, the (as yet unpublished) evaluation emphasised results analysis. An evaluator (Douthwaite) was consulted to assist in the design of a baseline survey. She worked with the programme team (led by Jana) to, initially, develop a logic model in order to clarify goals and help the team think about all factors affecting the health seeking behaviour of young people.

Although the model's aim is to simplify a complex reality, it helps planners and programme implementers appreciate this complexity when all the different risk and protective factors are listed – from individual psychosocial determinants to influences from partners, peers, parents, teachers and community. Before selecting the most important determinants, interviews were carried out with young people, parents, and community stakeholders such as teachers and service providers. This produced information on young people's use of time, patterns and processes of socialisation, places where they meet, substance abuse, and other crucially relevant information. The geographic mobility of girls emerged as an important issue affecting access to information and services. Young people also identified building self-esteem and confidence as major factors likely to influence the practice of safer sex. Further work with young people established that building confidence could be more suitably achieved by encouraging participatory activities, such as community service and cultural pursuits with local youth clubs, rather than by using the traditional strategy of organising life-skills workshops.

Young people were also asked to list sexual activities in order to access the colloquial terms used to describe them. This exercise initially shocked the project staff when they learned about the wide range of sexual activities known to young people. Some team members felt acutely uncomfortable, making each individual member reflect on his or her own moral stance. This led to an animated discussion within the team and offered the opportunity for clarifying the importance of being non-judgemental, respectful and open while talking to young people.

Throughout the planning process, the team members used an open and interactive system of discussion to analyse new information collected by team members. Discussions among the team members ranged from broad issues facing young people through to whether young people should be given contraceptives and to possible ways of sensitising service-providers to the needs of young people. This process of reflective data collection probably contributed the most in deciding intervention strategies.

The participatory planning process changed staff attitudes and challenged their assumptions. They became reflective and more attentive to the young people's lives. The needs assessment was thereby an intervention in itself as it started the mobilisation process throughout the community.

When designing interventions to improve the sexual health of young people, at least some research will be needed to ensure that strategies are appropriate to local circumstances and needs (McKay, 2000). The value of research at this stage, however, is often understated. Just how valuable it can be is highlighted in the following example from Vietnam. A contextual analysis conducted during the initial stages of the development of a life-skills approach in HIV education in schools found that students were interested in learning about sexual health, but that teachers felt unprepared to provide good quality sessions on sexual health. This initial research convinced officials at the Ministry of Education that action was needed and made them appreciative of young people's interest and concerns. The formal support of these officials and the partnership with teachers in developing the curriculum was crucial to the success of the programme (cited in Warwick and Aggleton, 2002).

Outcome evaluation and deciding on evaluation design

A programme based on an explicit theory of how activities relate to expected outcomes provides a roadmap for monitoring and evaluation (Lipsey, 1996; Weiss, 2004). For programme implementation, process and outcome evaluation, a completed logic model (see Figure 9.1) is read from the left, and shows what activities influence which determinants and hence behaviours and health outcomes.

To evaluate the impact of a programme, two basic questions must be addressed; namely, 'Can change be observed in the outcomes of interest?' and 'Can the observed change be attributed to the intervention?' Importantly, change should be measured at the population/community level, not just among those who participated in the programme.

The complexity and scale of intervention will determine at which level outcomes can be evaluated. Coombes (2004) has suggested that the pressure to demonstrate impact and account for funds spent has increased the interest in health status and behavioural outcomes as key 'evidence' of programme success. Yet single, time-limited small-scale interventions cannot realistically have a significant impact on individual behaviour or health status; nor from a health promotion perspective should these indicators be deemed the only measures of success. Changes in health behaviours and structural and environmental conditions occur over years, while changes in outcomes such as morbidity and mortality take even longer. If interventions are based on existing evidence or theory that the activities will have an impact on the determinants of young people's behaviour, their effectiveness should be assessed by measuring change in those determinants. If an intervention is shown to be effective in changing knowledge, skills, access to resources, or peer norms, then specific measures can be recommended for inclusion into more complex, longer-term, multi-level, multi-component interventions. In the latter case, success should be defined in terms of behavioural outcomes, and only in large-scale, multi-component programmes should biological end-points ever be evaluated (Ellis and Grey, 2004).

We briefly review below three main types of evaluation design – true experimental, quasi-experimental, and non-experimental designs (Fisher *et al.*, 2002). An important difference between these designs is the level of inference or attribution that can be made about the programme.

True experimental designs, such as randomised control trials (RCTs), are considered by some to be the only design that can demonstrate causality, or with confidence answer the question: 'Can the observed change be attributed to the intervention?'. In RCTs, often claimed to be the 'gold standard' or method of choice in outcome evaluations (Vitora *et al.*, 2004), individuals are allocated at random to the intervention or control group, and the two groups are compared. For interventions with young people delivered to schools, clinics or communities, it is rarely possible to completely exclude individuals from exposure to the programme. Instead, whole schools or communities are randomly assigned to receive the intervention or not. The purpose of random assignment is to ensure that the intervention and control group are truly comparable and differ only in their exposure to the intervention. Outcome indicators are measured at the start in a base line survey and later on in an end line survey. Any observed difference between the control and intervention group in outcome over time can therefore be attributed with more certainty, or greater probability, to the intervention (Ross and Wight, 2003; Coombes, 2004).

In the real world, however, the rigorous criteria necessary to implement RCTs or experimental evaluations pose practical challenges. For example, a randomised control trial designed to evaluate the MEMA *kwa Viijana* (Good things for young people) programme implemented in northern Tanzania encountered several hurdles. The programme aimed at improving the sexual health of young people and had four components – teacher-led and peer-assisted skills-based education in primary schools, provision of youth-friendly health services, condom social marketing by peers and raising community awareness and support (Wight and Obasi, 2003). However, unforeseen logistical problems arose throughout implementation that affected the feasibility of the intervention, and therefore the evaluation. These included the non-availability of classrooms, low levels of school attendance, irregular payment of teachers' salaries, and the small incentives – like free meals or a T-shirt – created envy and undermined the status of the peer educators. In this instance, the urgency to demonstrate success resulted in the intervention being evaluated too soon, and before real world implementation issues could be addressed (Wight and Obasi, 2003). In other situations, it may be difficult to isolate the control from the intervention group, or one or both from outside influences that may impact independently on programme outcomes. There may also be resistance to the use of comparison groups, particularly in resource poor settings, because of ethical concerns about withholding programmatic interventions from the young people in the control groups (Speizer et al., 2003). The implicit assumption underpinning such resistance, however, is that the intervention is a positive force, despite a lack of clear evidence.

Given these real world considerations, quasi-experimental designs may be more appropriate. Although the strength of evidence to demonstrate cause and effect is weaker than with experimental designs, most quasi-experimental designs still include a control group and provide *plausible* evidence that the programme produced the effect; that is, other explanations for the change can be largely discounted (Vitora et al., 2004). In some situations, however, such as communication programmes using the mass-media, it is near impossible to find an unexposed group that is similar to the exposed population. One solution to assess outcomes is to repeat cross-sectional surveys, as shown in the following example from Cameroon.

Here, the *100% Jeune* communication programme[1] targeted urban young people and urged them to use condoms consistently or to abstain from sex. This targeting was achieved through the mass media including television and radio-spots, a serial radio drama and call-in show, and a monthly youth newspaper. In addition, 20 peer educators reached 10,000 young people in- and out-of-school with interpersonal communication each month. Group sessions included role plays and skill-building exercises to negotiate abstinence and condom use. Two surveys, conducted 18 months apart, demonstrated an increase in several predictors/determinants of condom use targeted by the programme, including knowledge of a condom outlet, higher self-efficacy (less shy to buy condoms and more confident about using them correctly), and increased social support (higher perception of parental support for condom use, as well as increased discussion with friends regarding HIV and STIs). Respondents also reported higher condom use, but there was no change in the proportion having abstained from sex in the last year.

Can these trends be attributed to the *100% Jeune* programme or might they reflect a secular change? In the absence of a control group, Neukom and Ashford (2003) consider assessing the 'dose-response', or intensity of exposure, to different programme components. If those more exposed to the programme used condoms more and scored higher on predictors of condom use, it can be assumed that the programme is at least partly responsible for this trend. The evaluators defined high, medium, and low exposure to the programme, and analyses showed that higher exposure was associated with higher self-efficacy, perceived condom access, and discussion with friends about HIV. However, among young women, there was no difference in condom use according to exposure level, weakening the support that the positive trend in behaviour over the 18 months could be attributed to the programme. In a second evaluation a further 18 months later, however, condom use among women *was* associated with the level of exposure to the *100% Jeune* Programme (Plautz and Meekers, 2003).

While practical and logistical considerations pose particular challenges to implementing experimental evaluations, some claim that these designs are simply not appropriate for the evaluation of complex sexual health interventions aimed at behavioural and social change. In the real world, programmes operate in open systems and the evaluator has little control over many of these variations, many of which can influence the outcomes, challenging the internal validity of the study, and the generalisability of results (Lipsey and Cordray, 2000). Non-experimental evaluation with more emphasis on describing the programme's development in relation to the social context may be more suitable for providing valid results especially for more complex interventions (Potvin *et al.*, 2001). On the question of attribution of effect, programme theory as presented in a logic model is increasingly useful in the evaluation of complex programmes (Weiss, 2004). Weiss argues that if it can be shown that the programme moved along its expected sequence of steps, and that participants responded as hoped to each step, then it is reasonable to attribute observed change to the programme. Contextual information is important in understanding the complex and dynamic nature of local sexual cultures and how interventions operate within that context. Sexual behaviour carries meanings and is enacted in interpersonal, socio-cultural and historic contexts, and these meanings are fluid and change over time (Kippax and Van de Ven, 1998, and see Chapter 2 in this volume). For example, this is illustrated with the emerging protective practices among young people in Mozambique. For some young people, innovations in safer sex are associated with the practice of saca cena, or a one-night stand, linked to consistent condom use. In this context, traditional norms regarding sexual relationships are challenged with the overt expression of sexual power by young women combining sexual experimentation with responsibility and risk reduction (Karlyn, 2005).

The young people's programme implemented by CINI – outlined earlier – provides a useful example of how a programme can interact with the socio-cultural context and evolve. Baseline data conducted as part of the evaluation showed that a large proportion of young men (17 per cent) and women (33 per cent) were neither in school/college nor engaged in income-earning activities, and reported 'doing nothing'. Subsequent discussions with young people revealed the need to develop innovative ways to constructively engage them if they were going to benefit from the sexual health intervention. Activities such as linking them with other youth groups in the community, or encouraging participation in a village level campaign for cleaning ponds, were developed and later snowballed into a comprehensive approach wherein reproductive and sexual health did not remain the 'only focus', but became part of a broader development initiative. Thus, well into the implementation stage, even expected outcomes may change, which is perhaps not unusual given the iterative nature of projects committed to participation. Indeed 'there may be no predefined endpoint or criteria for a successful outcome' in some forms of community development work (Jewkes, 2004: 124) with obvious challenges for pre-planned outcome evaluation.

We stress here that strategies to evaluate the effects of different programmatic interventions cannot be standardised. Community-based programmes and community mobilisation programmes with a focus on empowerment and on changing the social environment young people live in, cannot be evaluated in the same way as improvements in treatment or counselling which are targeted at the individual (Jewkes, 2004). What is valued as an outcome of success in these two approaches will be different. In the first, since activities are directed towards enabling people to take action, participation and partnership are valued processes, and empowerment of individuals and communities are seen as valued outcomes (Nutbeam, 1998). Care should be taken to ensure that the evaluation itself does not compromise the integrity and effectiveness of a programme. If the measurement of outcomes dictates the aims of an initiative, there is a danger that outcomes and processes which are not easily quantifiable will be neglected, and that 'we will measure what is easily evaluable and ignore what is valuable' (Coombes and Thorogood, 2004: 5).

Meaningful outcome evaluations of programmes that aim to create a supportive environment for young people have not yet been conducted (Speizer *et al.*, 2003). In these complex programmes, more illuminative styles of evaluation are needed which describe and interpret the linkages between social structure and individual behaviours. The research designs for these kinds of evaluations tend to be descriptive rather than comparative (Patton, 1997).

In Ghana, community HIV/AIDS initiatives targeted young people and key adults concurrently to increase awareness about HIV and STIs and reduce stigma towards people living with HIV/AIDS. Both teachers and parents were encouraged to take an active part in sensitising young people on sexual health matters. Students who attended anti-AIDS clubs started requesting counselling and information on how to access sexual health services. Students and teachers alike reported being affected by testimonies of people living with HIV/AIDS and developed more positive attitudes towards them. Teachers trained in inter-generational communication skills reported changes in their own attitudes towards young people's concerns regarding sexual health, and felt more confident communicating with them. Parents who attended meetings – where two trained students facilitated a session on HIV/AIDS and STI – expressed a need for training in communication skills, so that they could talk more easily with their children (cited in Wood and Aggleton, 2003). This on-going evaluation demonstrates evidence of an increase in health literacy, improved social support and community competency to communicate about sexual health. It illustrates the processes of how health promotion outcomes and behavioural determinants change.

There is an increasing acceptance of methodological pluralism in evaluating health promotion. Whichever design is employed, evaluations – and therefore programmatic interventions – will improve by using rigour in information gathering and interpretation and taking a systematic approach as a priority over casual observation (Rootman *et al.*, 2001).

Using process evaluation to improve sexual health programmes

Typically, process evaluations address whether the intervention was implemented as planned in all areas, what proportion of the target population received the intervention, and in what form, what young people thought about the intervention, whether there were components they liked or disliked, and whether there were other factors that could influence the effect of the activities. A programme may not always reach all groups equally. In Rwanda, monitoring showed that young women made up only ten per cent of all clients at a youth centre which provided HIV counselling and testing and other sexual health services in a recreational and educational setting. Once opportunities for personal development were offered (such as skill-building courses in English, hairdressing, car mechanics and embroidery), 40 per cent of all the young people attending the centre were female, increasing the number seeking reproductive health services (Neukom and Ashford, 2003).

Whatever the evaluation design, monitoring the implementation of a programme is crucial and not optional. If a programme is not doing what it set out to do, effective monitoring can provide early feedback for the programme to course- correct. Keeping track of the coverage of a programme is also important. Theoretically, peer networks can have a wide reach, yet peer educators may fail to maintain contact with their peer groups. Routine programme information in the *100% Jeune* programme in the two cities in Cameroon (outlined above) indicated that initially 20 peer educators reached 10,000 young people each month. After 18 months, the extent of coverage was assessed in a community-based survey, with 12 per cent of young people having attended a peer education session. Only 5 per cent, however, had personally spoken to a peer educator; exposure to mass-media was obviously much higher, with 74 per cent of respondents in the survey having read a *100% Jeune* newspaper, 47 per cent having heard the call-in radio show, and 26 per cent reported following the radio drama during the previous three months. Peer educators may not always reach that many people, especially in longer-term interactive group interventions. It is not sensible to assess impact at the community level if process data show that the programme is poorly implemented or is targeting a very small audience. In the ideal world, programme managers together with funding agencies and evaluators should use process evaluation to decide whether impact assessment at community level is a wise investment of resources.

Detail on the implementation of the programme is also crucial to the interpretation of results of an outcome evaluation (Wight and Obasi, 2003; Coombes, 2004). Whatever the design, sufficient information on the intensity and frequency of intervention strategies is important in order to assess whether a similar programme in a different context might be successful (Ellis and Grey, 2004). Unfortunately, to date, few outcome evaluations of sexual health programmes aimed at young people have included details about implementation, leading some to comment that variations in outcome may be due to differences in programme management and supervision rather than the effectiveness of the intervention strategies (Speizer *et al.*, 2003; Erulkar *et al.*, 2004; Gallant and Maticka-Tyndale, 2004).

An absence of programme effect may also be due to an evaluation design, with insufficient statistical power to detect effects on behaviour. In a recent review of 11 evaluated school-based HIV prevention programmes in sub-Saharan Africa, lack of experimental effect was found to be due to poor evaluation design because of small sample sizes and/or possibly poor implementation of the programme. Because most interventions had failed to include a process evaluation – or had not been closely monitored – it was impossible to fully understand the reasons for the lack of effect (Gallant and Maticka-Tyndale, 2004).

Building the evidence base

As argued at the start of this chapter, policy makers and programme planners who set priorities and allocate resources want a synthesis of what is currently known to be the most promising intervention strategies. Systematic reviews of the evidence base often use strict criteria, including studies that measure at least behavioural outcomes and use 'rigorous' methodology. As pointed out in a review of reviews, summarising the evidence into the effectiveness of non-clinical interventions in the prevention of sexually transmitted infections, health promotion outcomes are often not fully reported (Ellis and

Grey, 2004). Without information on changes in determinants of risk, we cannot understand how and why an intervention is effective nor can we make assumptions about its transferability.When reviews exclude evaluations that only measure changes in determinants of risk much valuable information is lost, and effectiveness data from most reviews become inadequate for small-scale interventions (Ellis and Grey, 2004).

The dominance of, and exclusive reliance on, findings from experimental designs to assess effectiveness of health interventions severely restricts the knowledge base of what works (Black, 1996; Speller *et al.*, 1997; Nutbeam, 1999; Van de Ven and Aggleton, 1999; Merzel and D'Aflitti, 2003). The evidence will be skewed in favour of certain interventions (for example, teacher-led education versus community-based education) and certain population groups (Van de Ven and Aggleton, 1999). For example, a review of evidence base from interventions targeted at the most vulnerable young people (10 to 24-year-olds who engage in sex work, men who have sex with men, and injecting drug users) in developing countries set minimum criteria requiring at least a quasi-experimental design. No articles were found in peer-reviewed journals which measured a change in HIV risk behaviour (although 13 studies were identified in the grey literature) (Hoffman, 2006, personal communication). It is indeed far more difficult to reach and study these groups because of the illegal and/or stigmatised nature of the risk behaviour, but that does not mean that we have not learned very important programmatic lessons from working with these groups. The evidence base needs to be strengthened incrementally with small pieces of evidence adding up to a stronger case. We need not confuse small-scale and incremental evaluation with poor evaluation (Coombes, 2004).

Evaluation as intervention

The impact of evaluation comes not only from using the findings but from engaging in the evaluation process (Patton, 1997). Evaluation procedures help by developing knowledge that is valuable at the local level, and also contributes by developing skills that help individuals and community stakeholders take control of those factors affecting their health (Goodstadt *et al.*, 2001).

Participatory evaluation is a process controlled by the people in the programme or community. Participation increases the appreciation of the purpose of evaluation, understanding and acceptance of findings, and promotes commitment to act on them. The CINI example from India (outlined earlier) demonstrates that field staff easily developed their evaluation thinking skills resulting in greater focus on outcomes and openness for different ways to get there. They initiated an extensive and continued dialogue with the young people who, in turn, developed critical thinking skills and became architects of the programme. All this no doubt greatly improves the impact of the intervention, since the process of participation is itself believed to be health generating (Springett, 2001; Jewkes, 2004) and thus becomes a valued programme outcome. This example demonstrates that the main work and benefit of evaluation is at the grassroots level. There are, however, inherent conflicts between international information needs from evaluation focused on effectiveness, and those which inform and empower people at the local level (Patton, 1997). The credibility of participatory evaluation may still be challenged as insufficiently independent. Yet programmes evolve through interaction with their context, and it is the in-depth understanding of how programmes change and interact with the environment to reach their objectives and desired outcome that exemplifies the contribution of evaluation to improving the programme (Potvin *et al.*, 2001).

Conclusions – implications for research

The process of thinking about evaluation adds a much needed systematic rigour to the design of sexual health programmes for young people, and it introduces an opportunity to base design on theory, evidence, and community goals. Increasing attention is being placed on utilisation-focused evaluation and, most crucial for improving programmes, is that evaluation is a continuing iterative activity that includes monitoring and learning. Programmes evolve through interaction with their context, and research should gain in-depth understanding of this dynamic to interpret any changes in the outcomes. A range of methods is needed to evaluate multi-level and multi-component sexual health programmes, and evidence never comes from one study but is built incrementally by pooling results from a range of studies. Involving young people in both design and evaluation is health generating in itself, since it increases engagement in the programme and community goals, and enhances ownership.

Note

1   For futher information on the *100% Jeune* programme, see:
    www.100pourcentjeune.org/qui.html
    www.psi.org/where_we_work/cameroon.html
    www.ncbi.nlm.nih.gov/entrez/query.fcgi?cmd=Retrieve&db=PubMed&list_uids=15909360&dopt=Abstract

References

Black, N. (1996) Why we need observational studies to evaluate the effectiveness of health care, *British Medical Journal*, 312, 1215–18.
Chapman, S. (2004) Evaluating social marketing interventions, in M. Thorogood and Y. Coombes (eds) *Evaluating Health Promotion: Practice and methods*, Oxford: Oxford University Press, 93–109.

Coombes, Y. (2004) Evaluating according to purpose and resources: Strengthening the evidence base incrementally, in M. Thorogood and Y. Coombes (eds) *Evaluating Health Promotion: Practice and methods*, Oxford: Oxford University Press, 27–39.

Coombes, Y. and Thorogood, M. (2004) Introduction, in M. Thorogood and Y. Coombes (eds) *Evaluating Health Promotion: Practice and methods*, Oxford: Oxford University Press, 3–10.

DiClemente, R.J. and Wingood, G.M. (2003) Human immunodeficiency virus prevention for adolescents. Windows of opportunity for optimizing intervention effectiveness, *Archives of Pediatric and Adolescent Medicine*, 157(4), 319–20.

Ellis, S. and Grey, A. (2004) *Prevention of Sexually Transmitted Infections (STIs): A review of reviews into the effectiveness of non-clinical interventions*, London: Health Development Agency.

Erulkar, A.S., Ettyang, L.I.A., Onoka, C., Nyaga, F.K. and Muyonga, A. (2004) Behavior change evaluation of a culturally consistent reproductive health program for young Kenyans, *International Family Planning Perspectives*, 30(2), 58–67.

Fishbein, M. (2000) The role of theory in HIV prevention, *AIDS Care*, 12(3), 273–8.

Fisher, A.A., Foreit, J R., Laing, J., Stoeckel, J. and Townsend, J. (2002) *Designing HIV/AIDS Intervention Studies. An operations research handbook*, Washington: Population Council.

Gallant, M. and Maticka-Tyndale, E. (2004) School-based HIV prevention programmes for African youth, *Social Science and Medicine*, 58, 1337–51.

Goodstadt, M.S., Hyndman, B., McQueen, D.V., Potvin, L., Rootman, I. and Springett, J. (2001) Evaluation in health promotion: Synthesis and recommendations, in I. Rootman, M. Goodstadt., B. Hyndman, D.V. McQueen, L. Potvin, J. Springett and E. Ziglio (eds) *Evaluation in Health Promotion: Principles and perspectives*, Copenhagen: World Health Organisation, 517–33.

Hoffman, O. (2006 – personal communication).

Jewkes, R. (2004) Evaluating community development initiatives in health promotion, in M. Thorogood and Y. Coombes (eds) *Evaluating Health Promotion: Practice and methods*, Oxford: Oxford University Press, 123–34.

Karlyn, A.S. (2005) Intimacy revealed: Sexual experimentation and the construction of risk among young people in Mozambique, *Culture, Health and Sexuality*, 7(3), 279–92.

Kippax, S. and Van de Ven, P. (1998) An epidemic of orthodoxy? Design and methodology in the evaluation of the effectiveness of HIV health promotion, *Critical Public Health*, 8(4), 371–86.

Kirby, D. (2002) *BDI Logic Models: A useful tool for designing, strengthening and evaluating programs to reduce adolescent sexual risk-taking, pregnancy, HIV and other STDs* (available at <www.etr.org/recapp/BDILOGICMODEL 20030924.pdf>).

Kirby, D., Short, L., Collins, J., Rugg, D., Kolbe, L., Howard, M., Miller, B., Sonenstein, F. and Zabin, L. (1994) School-based programs to reduce sexual risk behaviours: A review of effectiveness, *Public Health Reports*, 109(3), 339–60.

Klein, M., and Coombes, Y. (2005) *Trust and Condom Use: The role of sexual caution and sexual assurances for Tanzanian youth (a baseline survey)*, Washington DC: Population Services International.

Lipsey, M. (1996) Key issues in intervention research: A program evaluation perspective, *American Journal of Industrial Medicine*, 29(4), 298–302.

Lipsey, M. and Cordray, D. (2000) Evaluation methods for social intervention, *Annual Review of Psychology*, 51, 345–75.

McKay, A. (2000) Prevention of sexually transmitted infections in different populations: A review of behaviourally effective and cost-effective interventions, *Canadian Journal of Human Sexuality*, 92, 95–120.

Merzel, C. and D'Afflitti, J. (2003) Reconsidering community-based health promotion: promise, performance and potential, *American Journal of Public Health*, 93(4), 557–74.

Neukom, J. and Ashford, L. (2003) *Changing Youth Behavior through Social Marketing: Program experiences and research findings from Cameroon, Madagascar, and Rwanda* (available at <www.psi.org/resources/pubs/PSIChangingBehavior.pdf >).

Nutbeam, D. (1998) Evaluating health promotion–progress, problems and solutions, *Health Promotion International*, 13(1), 27–44.

Nutbeam, D. (1999) Editorial: The challenge to provide 'evidence' in health promotion, *Health Promotion International*, 14(2), 99–101.

Odutolu O. (2005) Convergence of behaviour models for AIDS risk reduction in sub-Saharan Africa, *International Journal of Health Planning and Management*, 20(3), 239–52.

Patton, M.Q. (1997) *Utilization-Focused Evaluation: The new century text*, Thousand Oaks: Sage Publications.

Plautz, A. and Meekers, D. (2003) *Evaluation of the Reach and Impact of the 100% Jeune Youth Social Marketing Program in Cameroon*, Washington DC: Population Services International.

Potvin, L., Haddad, S. and Frohlich, K.L. (2001) Participatory approaches to evaluation in health promotion, in I. Rootman, M. Goodstadt., B. Hyndman, D.V. McQueen, L. Potvin, J. Springett and E. Ziglio (eds) *Evaluation in Health Promotion: Principles and perspectives*, Copenhagen: World Health Organisation, 45–62.

Rootman, I., Goodstadt, M., Potvin, L. and Springett, J. (2001) A framework for health promotion evaluation, in I. Rootman, M. Goodstadt., B. Hyndman, D.V. McQueen, L. Potvin, J. Springett and E. Ziglio (eds) *Evaluation in Health Promotion: Principles and perspectives*, Copenhagen: World Health Organisation, 7–38.

Ross, D.A. and Wight, D. (2003) The role of randomized controlled trials in assessing sexual health interventions, in J. Stephenson, J. Imrie and C. Bonell (eds) *Effective Sexual Health Interventions: Issues in experimental evaluation*, Oxford: Oxford University Press, 35–48.

Rothschild, M.L. (1999) Carrots, sticks, and promises: A conceptual framework for the management of public health and social issue behaviors, *Journal of Marketing*, 63, 24–37.

Speizer, I.S., Magnani, R.J., and Colvin, C.E. (2003) The effectiveness of adolescent reproductive health interventions in developing countries: A review of the evidence, *Journal of Adolescent Health*, 33(5), 324–48.

Speller, V., Learmonth, A. and Harrison, D. (1997) The search for evidence of effective health promotion, *British Medical Journal*, 315, 361–63.

Springett, J. (2001) Participatory approaches to evaluation in health promotion, in I. Rootman, M. Goodstadt., B. Hyndman, D.V. McQueen, L. Potvin, J. Springett and E. Ziglio (eds) *Evaluation in Health Promotion: Principles and perspectives,* Copenhagen: World Health Organisation, 83–105.

UN (2001) *Declaration of Commitment on HIV/AIDS,* United Nations General Assembly Special Session on HIV/AIDS, 25–27 June 2001, New York: United Nations.

Van de Ven, P. and Aggleton, P. (1999) What constitutes evidence in HIV/AIDS education? *Health Education Research,* 14, 461–71.

Vitora, C.G., Habicht, J-P. and Bryce, J. (2004) Evidence-based public health: Moving beyond randomized trials, *American Journal of Public Health,* 94(3), 400–5.

Warwick, I. and Aggleton, P. (2002) *The Role of Education in Promoting Sexual and Reproductive Health,* Safe Passages to Adulthood programme Knowledge Synthesis report, Southampton: Centre for Sexual Health Research, University of Southampton.

Weiss, C. (2004) On theory-based evaluation: Winning friends and influencing people, *The Evaluation Exchange,* ix(4), 2–3.

Wellings, K. and Macdowall, W. (2004) Evaluating mass media approaches, in M. Thorogood and Y. Coombes (eds) *Evaluating Health Promotion: Practice and methods,* Oxford: Oxford University Press, 145–61.

Wight, D. and Obasi, A. (2003) Unpacking the 'black box': The importance of process data to explain outcomes, in J. Stephenson, J. Imrie and C. Bonell (eds) *Effective Sexual Health Interventions: Issues in experimental evaluation,* Oxford: Oxford University Press, 151–66.

Wood, K. and Aggleton, P. (2003) *Stigma, Discrimination and Human Rights,* Safe Passages to Adulthood programme Knowledge Synthesis report, Southampton: Centre for Sexual Health Research, University of Southampton.

Chapter 10

Sexual health communication

Letting young people have their say

Wendy Macdowall and Kirstin Mitchell

Introduction

Reports on the sexual and reproductive health of the world's young people make for difficult reading; more than 10 million young people currently live with HIV/AIDS, around 100 million new cases of curable sexually transmitted infections (STIs) occur annually, and significant morbidity arises from complications of pregnancy and termination (UN, 2005). Less well documented, but just as disturbing, are the feelings of regret, shame, guilt, or exploitation that often accompany (too) early sexual activity. In response to the magnitude of this problem, young people, adults, authorities and institutions have employed various sexual health promotion strategies. Communication lies at the heart of such strategies, whether health education, social mobilisation or advocacy.

An understanding of the context in which young people send, receive and internalise (or decode) messages about sexual health is central to the design of effective communication strategies. Eaton and colleagues (2003), in a review of the factors that influence sexual behaviour among young people in South Africa, describe three domains of influence – namely, personal, proximate and distal contexts. Within the personal domain, knowledge and beliefs, perceptions of risk, and self-efficacy are the factors commonly focused upon by health programmes and interventions. But such personal factors represent only part of the picture; proximate interpersonal factors within sexual relationships, within friendship groups and between adults and children, significantly shape the nature of communication. Moreover, within a sexual relationship, imbalances of power created by gender, age or status are common (see Holland *et al.*, 1991 and other chapters in this volume for further discussion). The South African research suggests that many young women are in coercive male-dominated sexual relationships (Eaton *et al.*, 2003, and see Chapter 7 in this volume).

Even without such obstacles, communication can be tricky; we know many people find it difficult to talk openly about sex with a partner, and condoms tend to have negative connotations because suggesting their use implies infection or mistrust (Mitchell and Wellings, 2002, and Chapter 2 in this volume). Much has already been written about the influence of friendship groups, both positive and negative (for example, see Kobus, 2003). Friends play a crucial role in determining which messages get heard and how they are interpreted and acted upon. Power imbalances in adult-to-child communication also make young people particularly vulnerable to negative messages from parents and adults in authority. To take just one example, young people in a South African study reported being scolded or mocked by clinic staff when they asked for condoms (Eaton *et al.*, 2003).

At the environmental level, young people may lack access to information and services such as condoms and educational media (Eaton *et al.*, 2003). They may simply lack things to do in order to keep them from 'getting into trouble'. Distal cultural and structural factors also have a powerful influence on sexual behaviour (Eaton *et al.*, op. cit.). Importantly, young people often lack a voice with which to express their rights and needs, and they are sometimes viewed (by adults) as incapable of making the 'right' decisions. Young women, in particular, may be imbued (again by adults) with an innocence which requires protection (Aggleton *et al.*, 2004). These are the manifestations of the social and cultural 'rules' which govern the role of young people in society and the expression of their sexuality.

All cultures have social scripts regarding the sexuality of young people. These scripts define the parameters of what is acceptable and 'normal', and what is unacceptable and 'deviant'. In many cultures, there are different expectations of young men and young women in terms of acceptable behaviour, with tighter controls placed on young women (ostensibly to 'protect' them). Such restrictive scripts are shaped by adult fears of young people's sexuality and from the mistaken belief that talking about sex will encourage this sexuality to develop. Given this, it is unsurprising that there are few countries in the world where young people's sexual behaviour can be discussed openly and where prevention efforts have been met without some form of resistance or controversy.

This context provides a number of challenges for communication. The dominant belief that adults 'know what's best' for young people as regards their sexual health has meant that we have found it very difficult to genuinely let young people have their say and, when we do, there are sometimes negative ramifications. For instance, in South Africa, following consultation with young people, the Treatment Action Campaign's (TAC) programme to encourage young people to use condoms designed hard-hitting radio slogans such as 'Got no protection? Can't use your erection', 'Cloak the joker before your poker', 'Cover your vein, then drive her insane', 'Cuff your carrot before you share it' and 'No glove, no love'. Although young people identified with the messages, some (non-target) adult listeners complained (de Kock, 2005). Knowing how much of what sort of message to give at what stage is another key challenge. Age, though convenient, provides only an approximate indicator. Despite decades of formal and informal communication about sex, there is little in the way of non-partisan guidelines and value-free research to guide us.

While recognising that much communication about sexual matters takes place in the informal spheres of friends and family, this chapter focuses on planned and deliberate health communication strategies in more formal settings. Health communication has been defined as 'the study and use of methods to inform and influence individual and community decisions that enhance health' (Nelson *et al.*, 2002: 6). It derives from basic principles of communication concerning the transmission of messages from a sender to a receiver. Essentially, it is a 'hybrid' discipline that draws on a number of different specialties as diverse as the behavioural sciences and business studies (Nelson *et al.*, 2002).

The advent of HIV and AIDS has arguably affected the theory and practice of health communication more profoundly than any other issue (Flanagan *et al.*, 2001) and we now have a much better understanding of strengths and weaknesses of health communication, and the factors associated with a greater chance of success. In this chapter, we offer a brief overview of the changing emphasis in sexual health communication strategies since the late 1980s, highlighting three lessons in design – information in isolation can never be enough, theory is important but context is critical, and multi-layered approaches to communication are most effective. We then look at two different communication strategies in more detail – mass media and peer education.

Information alone is not enough to change behaviour

Early HIV/AIDS communications – so called IEC (Information, Education Communications) – tended to concentrate on the trilogy of knowledge, attitudes and behaviour, and were based on the premise that given the 'right' knowledge, individual attitudes would change, which in turn would lead to the required behaviour change. There is now universal consensus that this model is inadequate in reflecting the complexities of human behaviour, particularly sexual behaviour, and has limited scope in developing meaningful programmes that engage with young people in their everyday lives. The focus on individual responsibility, rather than the wider determinants of health, can result in victim blaming – 'we've told you what do to; it is your fault if you don't do it and so you will have to suffer the consequences' so the argument goes (Macdowall *et al.*, in press).

In the early 1990s, Behaviour Change Communication (BCC) largely replaced IEC as the strategy of choice. (Flanagan *et al.*, 2001). Implicit in this change of strategy was recognition that to promote behaviour change a different type of communication was needed. Unlike IEC, BCC explicitly recognised the role of theory and research in the development of interventions and sought to affect not just behaviour but the social context in which it occurred. In other words, practitioners in the field conceded that information alone was not enough.

Theory is important but context is critical

Theories of communication and behaviour change are helpful in creating appropriate message strategies and in choosing the right vehicles in which to place messages (Randolph and Viswanath, 2004). Communication strategies are commonly based on theories and models derived from the behavioural sciences. Taken together, these models highlight a number of important factors, as shown in Box 10.1.

These theories are useful in understanding and explaining sexual behaviour as well as in providing the building blocks for effective communication strategies. However, many of these theories derive from empirical research in Western settings and, it is argued, such theories 'are predicated on Western notions of individual autonomy and purpose' and 'may hold less relevance for populations in traditional communal cultures, where individual identity is grounded in family and community roles' (Elder, 2001: 16). In 1999, UNAIDS developed a new framework for HIV/AIDS communication which placed greater emphasis on the social and environmental context, as opposed to individual behaviour. It identified five domains of context as 'virtually universal factors in communications for HIV/AIDS preventive health behaviour' (UNAIDS/PennState, 1999). These are shown in Box 10.2.

Box 10.1

The different theories of behaviour change highlight:

- The importance of knowledge and beliefs about health
- The importance of self-efficacy: the belief in one's competency to take action
- The importance of perceived social norms and social influences related to the value an individual places on social approval or acceptance by different social groups
- The importance of recognising that individuals in a population may be at different stages of change at any one time
- The need to take account of socio-economic and environmental conditions
- The importance of shaping or changing the environment or people's perception of the environment

Source: Nutbeam and Harris (1999)

Box 10.2

The five contextual domains to focus on in developing communication strategies for HIV/AIDS communication strategies:

- Government policy – the role of policy and law in supporting or hindering interventions
- Socioeconomic status – the collective or individual income that may allow or prevent adequate intervention
- Culture – the positive, unique or negative characteristics that may promote or hinder prevention and care practices
- Gender relations – the status of women in relation to men in society and community and their influence on sexual negotiation and decision-making
- Spirituality – the role of spiritual/religious values in prompting or hindering the translation of prevention messages into health actions

Source: UNAIDS/PennState, 1999: 29–30

Within this framework, individual health behaviour is seen as a component of these domains, rather than the primary focus of health behaviour change.

Accepting that context is critical leads us naturally to the conclusion that communication strategies should seek to engender an environment that is as supportive as possible through methods such as advocacy, and community mobilisation. This leads us to our third point, which is that a multi-faceted approach is needed.

A multi-faceted approach is required

Mirroring developments in other areas of public health, the most recent shift in health communications has been towards a programmatic approach involving multi-component, multi-levelled interventions. Underpinning this strategy is a greater understanding of the wider determinants of health (many of which are beyond individual control). Family Health International (FHI) coined the term 'Strategic Behavioural Communication' (SBC) to describe this strategy, which replaced BCC in 2005. SBC is defined as:

> an interactive process with individuals and communities to develop tailored communications strategies, messages and approaches using a mix of communication channels and interventions to promote healthier behaviours and support individual community and societal behaviour change. It lends communication expertise to advocacy, social and community mobilisation and other interventions to deliver consistent

messages through multi-layered approaches and channels for maximum effectiveness.

(FHI, 2005: 5)

Programmatic interventions linked to this approach include peer education, counselling, support groups, mass media, traditional media, community mobilisation and advocacy, among others.

We now turn to look at two specific interventions in more depth; namely, mass communications and peer education. Both of these approaches have been used widely across the world in sexual health communications with young people, and both work best when the principles described above are rigorously applied. We draw predominantly on recent examples of HIV prevention among young people.

The mass media

It is universally acknowledged that the mass media are a powerful force for change (both positive and negative). The last few decades have seen rapid developments in communication technologies, which have resulted in new media channels being opened up to health promoters. The Internet and mobile phones are increasingly being used as media through which health-related messages may be transmitted. For example, a recent UK-based project sent text messages to young women, reminding them to take their contraceptive pill (see www.southbirminghampct.nhs.uk/_news/Press ReleaseLocal.asp?TitleID=501). In addition, satellite technology has resulted in the global reach of stations such as MTV.

The role of mass media in health can be considered in two different ways, as identified by Finnegan and Viswanath (1997); the first relates to the impact that day-to-day exposure to the media has on health outcomes while the second relates to the purposive use of the media to transmit health messages.

Research has explored the effects of day-to-day interaction with the mass media on a number of health-related behaviours in young people; for example, on violence, eating patterns, tobacco and alcohol use and, more recently, on sexual attitudes and behaviours (Escobar-Chaves et al., 2005). Studies have tended to focus on two main areas of concern: firstly, on the nature and extent of media consumption and its influence on attitudes and behaviour and, secondly, on the (often negative) media portrayal of health related behaviour and its influence on how people see the world (norm-sending). In recent years, the World Health Organisation (WHO) has begun to talk about a 'global youth media culture' driven by rapid advances in information and communication technologies:

Many of the daily perceptions, experiences and interactions that young people have are 'virtual', transmitted through various forms of information and entertainment technologies, the foremost of which continues to be television rather than Internet.

(WHO, 2004, www.un.org/esa/socdeu/unyin/
workshops/mediaculture-description.pdfture)

The effects of day-to-day interaction with the media are not all necessarily negative. We know that the media are an important source of information for many and that some of the messages portrayed are health-enhancing. Efforts have been, and continue to be, made to engage with programme makers (both TV and radio) and journalists to influence the way that sexual health issues are portrayed in the media (Macdowell *et al.,* in press).

Purposive use of the media involves utilising media channels to transmit messages, often using social marketing principles. Traditionally, this has involved high profile adverts on the TV, radio or in print media with the aim of changing knowledge, attitudes or behaviour. More recently, a range of other approaches has been used, including media advocacy and edutainment, and it is here that the boundaries between the effects of day-to-day interaction and purposive use of the media become blurred. In addition, young people themselves are influencing the information environment though youth media projects; these include a Young Journalists Group in Viet Nam, which directly involves 300 young people and reaches more than 30 million radio listeners, and *Little Masters,* a magazine produced by children under 15 years in China. The magazine's production involves 20,000 young people and reaches an audience of one million (Kinkade and Macy, 2003). Here we will explore principles and examples from two purposive approaches – mass media communications and edutainment.

Mass media communications

The appeal of mass communications is that a wide audience can be reached. This reach has been taken to unprecedented levels though global campaigns such as MTV's 2002 HIV/AIDS campaign *Staying Alive* which, it is estimated, reached just under 800 million homes across the world (Waszak Geary, 2005). The scale of intervention means that even if only one per cent of people watching are influenced by the messages, then a large number of people are still being reached. Mass communications are also potentially useful in trying to reach 'hidden' groups in the population; for example, young men who have sex with men, and who may not identify with more targeted interventions directed at adult 'gay' men.

Mass communications can put sexual health on the public agenda through getting people 'talking about it', and confer status and legitimacy on invisible or taboo issues such that it becomes more acceptable to discuss them in public. Mass communications can also contribute to legislative change by influencing policymakers' perceptions of a problem and exerting pressure for action (Stead and Hastings, in press). In mass communications, the key ingredients include getting the message heard and getting the message right, and, as with all health communications, it is important to try and influence the environment so that it is more supportive (Randolph and Viswanath, 2004).

Getting the message across

Getting the message across is the primary aim in mass communication interventions. This is conventionally achieved by buying media space but, increasingly, partnerships have been formed with media organisations. For example, South Africa's *loveLife* campaign (www.lovelife.org.za) extended the scale and scope of the mass media element of its campaign through a partnership with the South African Broadcasting Corporation, which provided radio and television airtime as well as co-production funding (UNAIDS, 2004).

Mass media approaches are often supplemented by other means of transmitting messages, such as the distribution of health education materials or the generation of news coverage in the 'free media', that is the newspapers, magazines, TV and radio coverage rather than advertising. Using the commercial mass media is expensive and even a short campaign can use up a large part of the budget set aside for preventive interventions. A valid aim is to promote coverage of the campaign by the free media (Wellings and Macdowall, 2000).

Getting the message right

Getting the message right is as important as getting it across. Message precision is dependent on listening to, and knowing, the target audience, and mass media work involves extensive formative research and pre-testing of materials. Such formative research should include an exploration of the media used by the target audience to find the effective and appropriate media channels. Formative research should include the non-target group as, given the sensitive nature of the topic, it is important to minimise the possibility of any backlash.

Supportive environments

As we have already seen, behaviour change is only possible where the environment is conducive to such change. Randolph and Viswanath (2004) point to the reciprocal relationship between structural changes and media coverage: 'Media attention can strengthen the supportive environment for forming community coalitions and also lending legitimacy for policy and environmental change' (Randolph and Viswanath, 2004: 426). An explicit objective of many mass media communications is to influence the social context and to create a favourable climate in which interventions can be received – 'edutainment' can be a useful tool here.

Edutainment

Edutainment involves designing and implementing programmes with the dual aims of entertaining and educating. The media channel can be television or radio programmes (soap operas, chat shows, phone-ins for example), films, music, websites or computer games. There are many examples of edutainment including Cote d'Ivoire's *SIDA dans la Cité* (AIDS in the City) (Shapiro *et al.*, 2003), India's weekly reality youth show *Haath se Haath Milaa* (Let's join hands) developed in partnership with the BBC World Service Trust, *Doordarshan* (the National Television Service) and The National AIDS Trust (www.bbc.co.uk/worldservice/trust/developmentcommunications/story/2005/11/051125_project-india.shtml), Brazil's *Malhação* (Working Out) and Nicaragua's *Sexto Sentido* (Sixth Sense), (www.puntos.org.ni/default.php) which reaches 80 per cent of 13 to 17 year olds in the country (UNAIDS, 2004). Two particularly well known examples are Radio Tanzania's soap opera *Twende na Wakati* (Let's go with the times) and South Africa's *Soul City*.

Soul City consists of a prime time television drama serial, a radio drama broadcast in nine African languages and print material. It has covered a range of social issues across the series but HIV/AIDS has been a main theme since it started in 1994. The audience of *Soul City* is young and it is estimated that the sixth series reached nearly five million 8 to 15-year-old South Africans via the television, and over two million via the radio (*Soul City*, 2005). The programme seeks to effect change at the individual level (for example, awareness, knowledge and attitudes), within the community (for example, local organisational policy and practice and connecting people to local services) and within society (for example, impact on public debate and policy). This approach acknowledges the dual roles of the mass media; firstly, as a channel for the dissemination of health information and, secondly, as a vehicle in itself that can be used to bring about change in society. A specific aim of the sixth series was to draw attention to the effect of HIV/AIDS on children and to engender caring and supportive behaviours towards those affected, especially children. The evaluation reported that parents who watched or listened to *Soul City* were significantly more likely to talk to their children about HIV and AIDS than those parents not exposed, and that there was a significant increase in the proportion of people who thought that the presence of AIDS in a family affects children (*Soul City*, 2005).

Tanzania's *Twende na Wakati* was a radio soap opera, broadcast in Swahili, twice a week from 1993 to 1999. The specific aim of the programme was HIV prevention, but family planning, economic development and other health issues were also addressed (Vaughan *et al.*, 2000). *Twende na Wakati*, unusually for most national media interventions, was evaluated using a quasi-experimental design (Vaughan *et al.*, 2000). In order to create a comparison group, the programme was not broadcast from one regional transmitter between 1993 and 1995. After 1995, *Twende na Wakati* was broadcast across the whole country and the first two years of programmes were transmitted in the comparison area; this provided the researchers with a chance to see if any effects of the programme were repeated in the comparison area. Surveys were conducted at yearly intervals in both areas. The results showed significant decreases in the number of sexual partners among men and women, an effect which was repeated in the comparison area when the programmes were transmitted after 1995. Increased condom use was also seen among sexually active respondents; again this effect was also seen in the comparison area after 1995. Behaviour change was found to be associated with increased self-perceived risk of contracting HIV/AIDS, increased self-efficacy in relation to preventing HIV/AIDS, interpersonal communication about HIV/AIDS and identification with and role modelling of the primary characters in the soap opera (Vaughan *et al.*, 2000).

Despite the widespread use of mass communication strategies in sexual health promotion, their use remains controversial in some quarters. It has been argued that such interventions are too expensive and divert resources away from the community level where they are really needed. Some have argued that many mass communications are about 'selling' health, rather than empowering choice, and therefore stand on shaky ethical ground (Tones and Green, 2004). As mentioned above, it is also argued that they tend to be used in the service of individual behaviour change rather than addressing the wider determinants of health, and that in this respect may simply serve the agendas of politicians keen to be seen to be doing something (Macdowall *et al.*, in press). Proponents of mass communication methods would agree that they should not be seen as a 'magic bullet', but rather as a useful tool in programmatic approaches to promoting the sexual and reproductive health of young people, which may also include interpersonal methods of communication, such as peer education.

Peer education

Peer education has been described as 'the teaching or sharing of health information, values and behaviours by members of similar age or status groups' (Sciacca, 1987). In practice, peer education programmes comprise strategies as diverse as counselling, teaching and service referral but the philosophy of peer-to-peer communication is common to all. As a method, peer education primarily seeks to effect change at the individual level; however, the method also has the potential to modify group-level norms or generate collective action to bring about policy change.

The advent of HIV/AIDS has seen a proliferation of peer-led HIV/AIDS programmes involving young people in developing countries. Settings vary from schools and colleges to informal youth projects and street-based outreach work. Here we draw on the lessons learned by one such programme: the *Baaba* project, which trained street youth from urban centres in Uganda (see Box 10.3). Ideally, peer education activities should be integrated into a multi-layered programme of HIV/AIDS prevention, care and treatment activities (such as HIV testing and support services, policy and advocacy campaigns, and therapeutic services for those with AIDS), with peer educators providing linkages across programme activities (UNAIDS, 1999).

Assumptions underlying peer education

As an HIV/AIDS prevention method, peer education is widely valued and accepted, which is a major reason why programme managers select it as a strategy (UNAIDS, 1999), hence reinforcing the reputation. Peer education has intuitive appeal but in fact robust evidence for its effectiveness is surprisingly lacking. The dearth of rigorous outcome evaluations means that

---

Box 10.3 The *Baaba* Project, implemented by GOAL Uganda.

Established in 2001 and operating in the major urban centres of Uganda, the *Baaba* project works in partnership with 12 organisations (NGOs) catering for the immediate and longer-term needs of street youth. Each organisation has around 10 to 20 peer educators (so-called *Baabas*, meaning respected older sibling in local dialect). *Baabas* run HIV/AIDS prevention clubs and small group sessions within their NGO, as well as undertaking street outreach work, distributing condoms to sexually active children and sharing information using drama, puppetry and sport. They are elected by their peers and supervised by a staff member within their NGO. GOAL Uganda provides capacity building support to each of the member NGOs, as well as working to improve youth-friendly sexual health services and undertaking advocacy work targeting local leaders, police, military and child rights advocates. The project objectives are as follows:

- to reduce the sexual and physical risks associated with the environments in which street children and street youth live
- to increase the capacity of member NGOs to effectively promote life-skills and sexual and reproductive health amongst staff and child beneficiaries, and to advocate on behalf of those infected and affected by HIV/AIDS
- to empower street children and street youth with the knowledge, skills, motivation and support to sustain existing safe sexual behaviour and change unsafe behaviour.

Abridged from Mitchell (2003)

many of the claims made for the method need to be seen as 'working hypotheses' rather than as evidence for effectiveness. Although the process data from which best practice guidelines (such as *How to create an effective Peer Education Project* [Flanagan and Mahler, 1996]) are generated provide important pointers, they cannot guarantee successful outcomes. This is, of course, no reason to discard the approach, but caution needs to be applied in assuming that peer education will be effective, regardless of how it is implemented. Below, we briefly discuss six common claims made for peer education, and review the evidence with reference to sexual health projects targeting young people in resource poor settings.

Claim 1 – Peer education approaches are effective at communicating health messages

Peer education works by formally exploiting naturally occurring information sharing and advice giving channels between young people's friendship groups. Peer networks often involve frequent, diverse and reciprocal interactions in which young people learn sharing, empathy and other social skills (Milburn, 1995). Young peer educators are regarded as effective and credible communicators with inside knowledge of their intended audience (UNAIDS, 1999). In general, similarity between senders and receivers is thought to enhance the persuasiveness of messages. In particular, young peer educators can relate well to peers who are experiencing similar struggles (Milburn, 1995).

Evidence suggests that peer educators tend to prefer contacts with peers who are most similar to themselves (Mitchell *et al.*, 2001; Wolf and Bond, 2002). Where peer educators are selected on the basis of their leadership/role model qualities, it follows that peers of lower status, or who are high risk-takers, will be least similar to them and may be less likely to sustain contact. Thus, accessibility to hard-to-reach groups may be more difficult than adult programme managers imagine. Peer educators may require additional support in accessing and approaching these groups. A study involving several youth peer education projects in Ghana (Wolf and Bond, 2002) indicated that young people in contact with peer educators who are similar with respect to age, sex, ethnicity and school status (in-school or out-of-school) were more likely to have engaged in HIV/AIDS protective behaviour in the previous three months. Although the authors suggested that the similarity between the peer educators and their contacts may have led to effective behaviour change, the cross-sectional design of the study did not enable them to attribute causality. Equally plausible, though less appealing, is the argument that, in establishing contacts with peers who were most similar to them, the peer educators were simply 'preaching to the converted'. This is a risk of the peer education approach that needs to be explicitly recognised.

It is also important to recognise that, under certain circumstances, young people may not trust the information they receive from their peers and may prefer their information on sexual health matters to come from respected and credible adults (Helgerson and Peterson, 1988; Cline and Engel, 1991). This should not be seen as a weakness of the method, but rather as an opportunity for adults and young people to work together to provide a multifaceted approach, involving both young people and adult educators.

Claim 2 – Peer educators provide positive role models and benefit themselves from their role

Evidence suggests that the method benefits peer educators themselves, through the responsibility, recognition and skills enhancement conferred by the role (HEA, 1993; Phelps *et al.*, 1994; Wilton *et al.*, 1995). This was borne out by the *Baaba* project, with the peer educators often becoming 'leaders' with responsibilities far wider than HIV/AIDS education. A risk associated with these benefits, however, is that peer educators may use their position to exert inappropriate levels of influence over their peers. In the *Baaba* project, this risk was increased where NGO staff expected the *Baabas* to exert discipline and control over other (usually younger) children in the NGO (Mitchell, 2003).

It has been argued that peer educators serve as role models for their peers (Perry and Sieving, 1993), and that expectations of exemplary behaviour by other young people and programme managers may, in turn, impact positively on the behaviour of peer educators. It is also possible for peer educators to fall visibly short of expectations. For example, when a female *Baaba* became pregnant to a male *Baaba,* the implication that these two *Baabas* had failed to 'practice what they preach' had a negative impact on the target audience (Mitchell, 2003).

The extent to which peer educators benefit from the role may depend on who they are and how they are selected. Ebreo and colleagues (Ebreo *et al.*, 2002) found that young people chosen by their teachers because they were risk takers did not benefit significantly from being peer educators. They found that the risk takers were not credible to their peers with regard to risk reduction, did not work particularly well with classroom teachers and were not involved enough in school activities to be effective. Based on these findings, they recommend that peer educators should be motivated by altruistic reasons and selected by their classmates as being credible and competent.

Claim 3 – The approach is participatory and empowering

One of the appeals of peer education is that peer educators may be empowered (have power to take decisions in matters relating to themselves) through participation in the implementation of the project. Participation exists on a continuum – at one end, peer educators may simply follow a syllabus and teaching method pre-determined by adults while, at the other end, peer educators may be given responsibility for designing and implementing the entire range of activities. However, it is important to bear in mind that even the most participatory programmes essentially impose an 'adultist' agenda (such as prevention of teenage pregnancy or STIs) on the work of the peer educators (Milburn, 1995). Furthermore, regardless of the strategy, the extent to which a peer-led intervention is participatory depends on how much the adults involved in the programme are genuinely willing to hand over control. It is equally important to think critically about *who* is empowered; ensuring effective participation by the target audience is far more challenging than ensuring empowerment for peer educators, yet the former are the very young people who may benefit most from inclusion in project decisions.

It cannot be taken for granted that, as peer educators, young people will be less judgemental and more empathic than adults. Without adequate training and support, peer educators may end up simply transmitting the internalised attitudes, norms and beliefs of the adults in authority around them. In the *Baaba* project, *Baabas* sometimes chose to employ the didactic style of teaching customary to learning settings in Uganda. Having 'handed over' responsibility for teaching to the *Baabas,* the project had to carefully balance respect for this decision with encouragement towards more participatory teaching styles.

Claim 4 – Ongoing contact effectively reinforces messages

The importance of reinforcing positive messages is argued by social learning theory. Peer education has the potential to reinforce socially learned behaviour through the many opportunities a peer educator has to influence, persuade, teach and counsel peers (Jay *et al.*, 1984; Kelly *et al.*, 1991). The opportunity for ongoing reinforcement of positive messages is considerable, particularly where the peer educator is tasked with influencing members of his/her usual social group. In practice, not all youth-led sexual health programmes exploit this potential, with many projects relying on one-off sessions or highly structured inputs (Tudiver *et al.*, 1992; Phelps *et al.*, 1994). In other programmes, high turnover of peer educators and/or their target audience has diminished the potential for reinforcing messages.

Peer education also has the potential to address wider environmental determinants of behaviour as well as individual factors. But programme managers may need to be prepared to take the project well beyond the original narrow scope of HIV/AIDS or STI prevention. The *Baaba* project for instance, sought to address the negative attitudes of adults with responsibility for the protection of street children (such as Child Rights Advocates and the police) through a series of training days. Although ostensibly concerned with protecting street children from HIV/AIDS, the training days, in which the *Baabas* gave testimonies and performed role plays, proved to be powerful mechanisms in breaking down the widespread prejudice of security personnel towards young people on the street.

Claim 5 – The strategy backed up by theory

Peer education is said to have roots in three well-known theories (Milburn, 1995): social learning theory (Bandura, 1977, 1986) emphasising modelling as an important aspect in learning; social inoculation theory (Duryea, 1983) emphasising the potential negative influence of social and peer pressure on health behaviour; and differential association theory (Sutherland and Cressy, 1960) drawing on criminology research to posit that the skills, attitudes and motivations are learned through association with more experienced individuals in small peer groups. Although such theories provide a broad framework of justification, they offer only limited explanation for the effectiveness of peer education strategies (Milburn, 1995; Turner and Shepherd, 1999). In practice, peer education programmes adopt a diverse range of strategies which are seldom grounded in theory (Turner and Shepherd, 1999). Instead, 'working hypotheses and intuitively appealing concepts' tend to be conflated with basic theory (Milburn, 1995: 408). This has led some to describe peer education as 'a method in search of a theory' (Turner and Shepherd, 1999: 235).

Claim 6 – Peer education is cheaper than other methods

Peer education is popular among programme managers because the reliance on young unpaid volunteers to implement the main part of the programme is thought to be cost effective (UNAIDS, 1999). Cost-effectiveness studies have been largely confined to US-based projects and their estimates have varied, depending on the effectiveness of the strategy and variables, such as the existing prevalence of sexual health morbidity. Some strategies in some settings have reported cost-savings; for instance, in switching from health clinic based sexual health education to a peer outreach model in Mexico (Townsend *et al.*, cited in Senderowitz, 1997). Certainly, it is cheaper to use young volunteers than paid professionals to impart information, but this does not usually negate the need for intensive involvement by trained and committed staff (Milburn, 1995). Cost-effectiveness cannot be taken for granted as inherent to the method but must be sought via effective implementation and judicious use of resources.

Summary

Globally, the sexual and reproductive health status of young people is of grave concern. Communication strategies are an essential part of the strategy in responding to this public health issue. We know that information alone is not enough to change behaviour. We also know that an understanding of the context of communication is as important – if not more so – than adhering to any behavioural or communication theory. The context in which young people think about and engage in sexual activity makes them particularly vulnerable; inherent power imbalances and lack of available scripts serve to increase this vulnerability. Mass media and peer education are two types of communication approach which, if used as part of a multi-faceted approach, can effect positive change in individual attitudes and behaviour and the social norms in the wider community. The mass media also has a powerful function in setting the agenda which can, in turn, influence policy. Their effectiveness cannot be taken for granted, however; programmes and interventions that are responsive to the context in which communication takes place and which attempt, as far as possible, to let young people have their say, have a greater chance of success.

References

Aggleton, P., Chase, E. and Rivers, K. (2004) *HIV/AIDS Prevention and Care among Especially Vulnerable Young People: A framework for action*, Safe Passages to Adulthood/WHO, Southampton: Centre for Sexual Health Research, University of Southampton.

Bandura, A. (1977) *Social Learning Theory*, Englewood Cliffs, NJ: Prentice-Hall.

Bandura, A. (1986) *Social Foundations of Thought and Actions: A social cognitive theory*, Englewood Cliffs, NJ: Prentice-Hall.

Cline, R. and Engel, J. (1991) College students' perception of sources of information about AIDS, *Journal of the American College of Health*, 40, 55–63.

De Cock, C. (2005) Mixed reaction to new TAC condom campaign, *The Cape Argus*, 10 February, 2005.

Duryea, E. (1983) Using tenets of inoculation theory to develop and evaluate a preventive alcohol education intervention, *Journal of School Health*, 53, 250–6.

Eaton, L., Flisher, A. J. and Aarø, L. E. (2003) Unsafe sexual behaviour in South African youth, *Social Science and Medicine*, 56, 149–65.

Ebreo, A., Feist, S., Siewe, Y. and Zimmerman, R. (2002) Effects of peer education on the peer educators in a school-based HIV prevention program: Where should peer education research go from here? *Health Education and Behavior*, 29(4), 411–23.

Elder J.P. (2001) *Behaviour Change and Public Health in the Developing World*, London: Sage.

Escobar-Chaves, S.L., Tortolero, S.R., Markham, C.M., Low, B.J, Eitel, P. and Thickstun, P. (2005) Impact of the media on adolescent sexual attitudes and behaviours, *Paediatrics*, 116, 303–26.

Family Health International (2005) *Strategic Behavioural Communication (SBC) for HIV and AIDS: A framework,* Arlington: FHI.

Finnegan, J.R. Jr. and Viswanath, K. (1997) Communication theory and health behavior change, in K. Glanz, F.M. Lewis and B.K. Rimer (eds) *Health Behaviour and Health Education 2nd edition,* San Francisco: Jossey-Bass, 313–41.

Flanagan, D. and Mahler, H. (1996) *How to Create an Effective Peer Education Project: Guidelines for prevention projects,* Arlington VA: AIDSCAP/FHI.

Flanagan, D., Mahler, H. and Makinwa, B. (2001) Creating and applying a tool for upgrading behaviour change skills on-the-job, in B. Makinwa and M. O'Grady (eds) *Best practices in HIV/AIDS Prevention Collection,* Arlington VA/Geneva: FHI/UNAIDS.

HEA (1993) *Peers in Partnership: HIV/AIDS education with young people in the community,* London: Health Education Authority.

Helgerson, S. and Peterson, L. (1988) Acquired Immunodeficiency syndrome and secondary school students: Their knowledge is limited and their want to learn more, *Pediatrics,* 81, 350–5

Holland, J., Ramazanoglu, C., Scott, S., Sharpe, S. and Thomson, R. (1991) Between embarrassment and trust: Young women and the diversity of condom use, in P. Aggleton, P. Davies and G. Hart (eds) *AIDS: Responses, Interventions and Care,* Basingstoke: Falmer Press.

Jay, M., DuRant, R., Shoffitt, T., Linder, C. and Litt, I. (1984) Effect of peer counsellors on adolescent compliance in use of oral contraceptives, *Pediatrics,* 73,126–31.

Kelly, J., St., Lawrence, J., Diaz, Y., Stevenson, L., Hauth, A., Brasfield, T., Kalichman, S., Smith, J. and Andrew, M. (1991) HIV risk behaviour reduction following intervention with key opinion headers of population: An experimental analysis, *American Journal of Public Health,* 81, 168–71.

Kinkade, S. and Macy, C. (2003) *What works in Youth Media: Case studies from around the world,* Baltimore MD: International Youth Foundation.

Kobus, K. (2003) Peers and adolescent smoking, *Addiction,* 98 (suppl.1), 37–55.

Macdowall, W., Head, R. and Wellings, K. (in press) Mass Media Campaigns, in W. Macdowall, C. Bonell and M. Davies (eds) *Health Promotion Practice,* Maidenhead UK: Open University Press.

Milburn, K. (1995) A critical review of peer education with young people with special reference on sexual health, *Health Education Research,* 10, 407–20.

Mitchell, K. (2003) *The Baaba Project: Challenges and lessons learned,* unpublished report, Kampala: GOAL Uganda.

Mitchell, K. and Wellings, K. (2002) The role of ambiguity in sexual encounters between young people in England, *Culture, Health and Sexuality,* 4(4), 393–408.

Mitchell, K., Nakamanya, S., Kamali, A. and Whitworth, J. (2001) Community-based HIV/AIDS education in rural Uganda: Which channel is most effective? *Health Education Research,* 16(4), 411–23.

Nelson, D.E., Brownson, R.C., Remington, P.L. and Parvanta, C. (2002) *Communicating Public Health Information effectively. A guide for practitioners,* Washington DC: American Public Health Association.

Nutbeam, D. and Harries, E. (1999) *Theory in a Nutshell,* Sydney: McGraw Hill.

Perry, C. and Sieving, R. (1993) *Peer Involvement in Global HIV/AIDS Prevention Among Adolescents,* unpublished report commissioned by the Global Programme on AIDS, Geneva: World Health Organisation.

Phelps, F., Mellanby, A., Crichton, N. and Tripp, J. (1994) Sex education: The effect of a peer programme on pupils (aged 13–14 years) and their peer leaders, *Health Education Journal*, 53, 127–39.

Randolph, W. and Viswanath, K (2004) Lessons learnt from public health mass media campaigns: Marketing health in a crowded media world, *Annual Review of Public Health*, 25, 419–37.

Sciacca, J. (1987) Student peer health education: A powerful yet inexpensive helping strategy, *The Peer Facilitator Quarterly*, 5, 4–6.

Senderowitz, J. (1997) *Reproductive Health Outreach Programs for Young Adults*, Washington DC: FOCUS on Young Adults Research Series.

Soul City (2005) *Evaluation of Soul City Series 6*, Institute for Health and Development Communication, Houghton South Africa: Soul City (available at <www.soulcity.org.za>).

Stead, M. and Hastings, G. (in press) Media Advocacy, in W. Macdowall, C. Bonell and M. Davies (eds) *Health Promotion Practice*, Maidenhead UK: Open University Press.

Sutherland, E. and Cressy, D. (1960) *Principles of Criminology*, Philadelphia: Lippincott.

Tones, K. and Green, J. (2004) Mass communication and community action, Chapter 8 in *Health Promotion Planning and Strategies*, London: Sage, 240–68.

Turner, G. and Shepherd, J. (1999) A method in search of a theory: Peer education and health promotion, *Health Education Research*, 14, 235–47.

Tudiver, F., Myers, T., Kurtz, R., Orr, K., Rowe, C., Jackson, E. and Bullock, S. (1992) The talking sex project: Results of a randomized trial of small-group AIDS education for 612 gay and bisexual men, *Evaluation and the Health Professions*, 15, 25–42.

UN (2005) *World Youth Report 2005*, New York: United Nations.

UNAIDS (1999) *Peer Education and HIV/AIDS: Concepts, uses and challenges*, Geneva, UNAIDS.

UNAIDS (2004) *The Media and HIV/AIDS: Making a difference*, Geneva: UNAIDS.

UNAIDS/PennState (1999) *Communications Framework for HIV/AIDS: A new direction*, Geneva: UNAIDS.

Vaughan, P.W., Rogers, E.M., Singhal, A. and Swalehe, R.M. (2000) Entertainment-Education and HIV/AIDS Prevention: A field experiment in Tanzania, *Journal of Health Communication*, 5(Suppl.), 81–100.

Waszak Geary, C. (2005) *MTV's Staying Alive 2002 HIV Prevention Campiagn. YouthNet Brief No 2*, Arlington PA: YouthNet (available at <www.fhi.org/youth net>).

Wellings, K. and Macdowall, W. (2000) Evaluating mass media approaches to health promotion: A review of methods, *Health Education*, 100(1), 23–32.

Wilton, T., Keeble, S., Doyal, L. and Walsh, A. (1995) *The Effectiveness of Peer Education in Health Promotion: Theory and practice*, Bristol: Faculty of Health and Community Studies, University of the West of England.

Wolf, C. and Bond, K. (2002) Exploring the similarity between peer educators and their contacts and AIDS-protective behaviours in reproductive health programmes from adolescents and young adults in Ghana, *AIDS Care*, 14(3), 367–73.

WHO (2004) *Report of the Workshop on Global Youth Media Culture*, Geneva: World Health Organisation.

Chapter 11

Young people and sex and relationships education

Nicole Stone and Roger Ingham

Introduction

> The question is not whether children will get AIDS and sexual educa-
> tion, but how and what kind they receive. It is impossible to hide
> children from sexual influences. Adult role models, television, adver-
> tisements, parents and family bombard young children with them ...
> Silence and evasiveness are just as powerful teachers as a discussion of
> the facts.
>
> (McNab, 1981: 22)

Other chapters in this book illustrate how the contexts and environments in
which some young people live render them especially vulnerable to negative
physical and psychological sexual health outcomes. Young people across
the world, however, do not form an homogenous group and have diverse
needs, realities, preferences and vulnerabilities. Many grow up in relative
safety, unaffected by sexual exploitation, untouched by national or regional
conflict, and so on. While special attention certainly needs to be directed
towards those in especially vulnerable contexts (and, indeed, those who
enable and maintain such contexts), the provision of appropriate mainstream sexual health programming should not be overlooked, nor its
importance underestimated. To a large extent, all young people are vulnerable simply by virtue of their age and the ways in which many people in
positions of responsibility restrict their access to information and services.

There has been frequent and heated debate – for many years and in many
countries – concerning the most appropriate ways to address issues of sexual development. Topics of such debates have included the
age-appropriateness of sex and relationships education, whose responsibility it is, what should be covered, the most suitable style of delivery, the
extent to which approaches should be framed within specific religious
and/or cultural discourses and, indeed, whether such forms of education
should take place at all. This chapter discusses some of these issues, but
with a particular focus on poorer country contexts.

The changing sexual worlds of young people

Whether or not adults find it acceptable, many young people throughout the world engage in sexual activities. Ali and Cleland's chapter in this volume points to the changes that are occurring in the countries of sub-Saharan Africa and in Central and South America, and similar changes have been reported in many richer countries (Bozon and Kontula, 1998). In Asia, reported sexual activity outside of marriage has been found to be less prevalent (especially for young women) than in other settings, but a review of 34 studies, sponsored by the UNDP/UNFPA/WHO/World Bank Special Programme of Research Development and Research Training in Human Reproduction, revealed reported rates of activity in the 2–11 per cent range among unmarried young people, with wide gender disparities (Brown *et al.*, 2001).

Despite the challenges of getting accurate data on early sexual activity, there seems to be little doubt that changes are occurring among young people, and that more is happening earlier than in previous generations (although the paucity of research into sexual activity prior to the onset of HIV/AIDS makes long-term trends difficult to identify with any certainty). There are various reasons why these changes are occurring; among these are the general trend in most countries towards an increasing age of marriage coupled with reduction in the age of menarche, leading to a longer period of potential sexual activity outside of regular relationships (although these by no means guarantee safety from risk), increased exposure to global media (including the Internet) leading to greater exposure to more sexual content, internal migration from rural to urban settings, thereby removing some young people from their traditional forms of social (and sexual) control, and others.

It is not necessary to hold strong religious and moral beliefs to be concerned about these trends. While some may argue that there are no *a priori* reasons as to why young people should not explore and enjoy their emerging sexuality, a public health approach demands concern. There are a number of negative physical and psychological outcomes associated with early sexual activity that simply can not be ignored. These include unintended physical outcomes, such as pregnancy and sexually transmitted infections (STIs), as well as evidence that much early sexual activity is characterised by coercion and pressure (including from male to female, from older to younger, from media and peer pressure and so on) which may lead to subsequent regret and lowered self-esteem. Furthermore, in many contexts, pressures to fit societal norms of heterosexuality lead to immense difficulties for those who prefer not to follow that particular route (see also the Chapter 6 in this volume). A sexually healthy society or culture would be characterised by absence of unintended physical outcomes, positive psychological outcomes of sexual activity, high levels of mutuality and respect both in relation to partners and to the variety of sexual preferences and, although this is seldom discussed in policy and programmatic (or even academic) deliberations, some recognition of the role of pleasure (Ingham, 2005).

But reactions to such changing behavioural patterns, and views on the best ways to achieve sexually healthier societies, vary considerably. To put the matter simply, there are two competing discourses that recur with increasing regularity in many countries, and at many levels within countries from the highest level of political debate through to local gatekeepers in schools and health services, in communities and in families. Some believe that sex and relationships education increases the extent of experimentation and risk-taking, while others believe that education protects against negative outcomes. Following from these positions, some maintain that narrow religiously based encouragement to abstain from sexual activity (with the corollary that young people therefore will not need any information on contraception and so on) is to be preferred, while others believe that more open and comprehensive approaches are likely to lead to improved health outcomes. Of course, there are various intermediary positions within these two extremes, but it is probably true to say that the vast majority of people in positions of influence (which includes politicians, other policy-makers, parents, school governing bodies, and others) are pulled more strongly towards one pole than the other.

Attempts to resolve which of these approaches offers the greater chance of success have been generally based on two forms of approach: those involving rights-based approaches (for their own sake as well as to confront the 'righteous' claims of the 'moral right'), and those drawing on the available research evidence, limited though it may be.

Rights-based approaches

It is accepted (almost) globally that young people have a number of fundamental rights; these are enshrined in the UN Convention of the Rights of the Child (CRC) which has been ratified by all governments of the world with the exception of the USA and Somalia. The 'child' in this convention applies to all those aged up to 18 years. Included among the specific coverage are the rights to enjoyment of the highest attainable standard of health (Article 24), to education directed towards the development of personality, talents and mental and physical abilities to their fullest potential (Articles 28 and 29), to education and information including that relating to sex and sexual health matters (Articles 13 and 28) and to be free from any forms of sexual exploitation (Articles 34 and 36) (UN, 1989). In addition to the UNCRC, the international agreement covering the rights of women to be free from violence (UN, 1993) is clearly of direct relevance to the contexts of young people's sexual activity (see Chapter 7 in this volume), and the two International Conferences on Population and Development, held in Cairo in 1994 (UN, 1994) and New

York (UN, 1999) five years later, both placed great emphasis on the needs of 'adolescents'.

Similarly, UNAIDS has called for a series of initiatives to support young people in the light of the threat of HIV; these include creating a supportive environment, reaching those who influence young people, placing young people at the centre of the response, mobilising the educational system, mainstreaming HIV prevention and AIDS care for young people into other sectors, addressing gender inequalities, and opening dialogue on sensitive issues (UNAIDS, 2004).

So, from a number of rights-based perspectives, increased information and education is seen as an entitlement of young people, and there are obligations on national governments to implement programmes to support activities along these lines. However, strong opposition still remains in many parts of the world, and so it is additionally useful to consider the extent to which research evidence supports particular approaches to the area. This is an essential element in the pursuit of progress to improving the sexual health of young people.

The research evidence

As mentioned above, one of the main barriers to the promotion of sex and relationships work (including education) is the fear that talking to young people about sex related matters will encourage them to participate in it. Such anxieties can lead to, at the extreme, complete silence or, alternatively, they can – and generally do – encourage an over-emphasis on the negative (for example, unplanned pregnancy and STIs) rather than the positive aspects of sex (such as intimacy and pleasure). Such imbalanced approaches run the risk that young people may reject much of what adults have to say on the area, thereby leading them to seek guidance from less reliable or credible sources instead, such as peers and the media.

Evaluating the impact of one specific sexual health intervention is no easy task. Given the complexity of the factors that affect outcomes, it is unlikely that any one approach will have clearly measurable effects. Nevertheless, many researchers have indeed attempted to assess impacts, using a mix of methods ranging from the results of randomised control trials (the so-called Gold Standard) through to qualitative small-scale studies, and focusing on processes as well as outcome measures. This is not the place to discuss the relative merits of the different approaches; instead, a selective summary of some key findings is provided, drawn from studies carried out in different nation settings.

Research examining the effects of talking to young people about sexual matters on their behaviour offers no backing to the argument that it accelerates the onset of sexual experience or increases sexual risk-taking (Franklin *et al.*, 1997; Kirby, 1997, 2001, 2002abc; Family Health

International, 2002). Indeed, many studies from across the world show that good quality programmes can actually delay the onset of first sex and increase safer sexual practices. For instance, in 1997 a review of HIV and sexual health education programmes commissioned by the Department of Policy, Strategy and Research of UNAIDS, examined 68 reports on sexuality education from France, Mexico, Switzerland, Thailand, the UK, the USA, and various Nordic countries. Of the 53 papers which reported on the evaluation of specific interventions (in tertiary education institutions, clinical settings, by mail distribution and through public campaigns and community groups), 22 reported that the educational programme either delayed the onset of sexual activity, reduced the number of sexual partners and/or reduced unplanned pregnancy and STI rates. The review found minimal evidence to suggest that education about sexual health and/or HIV increased sexual activity; with only three studies finding increases in sexual behaviour associated with the education received (UNAIDS, 1997; Grunseit *et al.*, 1997). The authors concluded that there was 'little evidence to support the contention that sexual health and HIV programming promotes promiscuity' (UNAIDS, 1997: 6).

In 1997, and then again in 2001, Kirby and colleagues reviewed the research evidence from US and Canadian school-based programmes to show which, if any, can delay sexual initiation, increase contraceptive use and/or reduce unplanned pregnancy. Only studies meeting specific criteria, illustrating scientifically valid evidence, were included in the reviews. Findings showed that the most effective sex and relationships programmes delivered in schools shared ten common characteristics including: the delivery and reinforcement of clear messages; the provision of basic, accurate information about risks; ways to avoid intercourse and methods of protection; offered skills training; used a participatory approach; were delivered by dedicated, enthusiastic and trained adults or peer-leaders; and addressed social pressures. Furthermore, short-term programmes and those delivered in less than a few hours were not shown to have a measurable impact (Kirby, 1997, 2001). The extent to which Kirby's conclusions can be expected to be valid in countries with less well-established educational systems, however, is not clear.

Other assessments of the impact of the different approaches include a comparison of the situations in a number of developed countries; their report concludes that:

> ... where young people receive social support, full information and positive messages about sexuality and sexual relationships, and have easy access to sexual and reproductive health services, they achieve healthier outcomes and lower rates of pregnancy, birth, abortion and STDs.
>
> (AGI, 2001: 6)

Further support for the general approach is drawn from the UNICEF Report Card for 2001. Again assessing the situation in relation to teenage births in almost 30 of the richer countries in the world, the report concludes:

> This commentary has stressed throughout that success in lowering teenage birth rates is a matter of both motivation and means ... means – availability of contraception and education to enable informed and mutually respectful choices ... motivation – ... a stake in the future, a sense of hope, and an expectation of inclusion in an economically advanced society ...
>
> (UNICEF, 2001: 25)

What this same report stresses, in addition to the need for suitable education and services provision (the 'means'), is the importance of the wider economic context in affecting sexual activity and pregnancy choices (the 'motivation'). A similar issue was raised in Kirby's reviews, mentioned earlier; that schemes developed to support young people in more general ways than simply improving sex and relationships education had highly beneficial effects on outcomes.

Additional best practice guidelines, which have been identified through research, also include the desirability of providing sex and relationships programmes from an early age – ideally prior to the onset of sexual activity – and the importance of placing activities within the broader context of young people's lives. Research has shown that it can be easier to establish safe behaviour from the very outset of sexual involvement rather than changing established behaviours; hence, programmes aimed at sexually inexperienced young people have a critical role to play in the promotion of positive sexual health. Further, although appreciation of diversity and the conveyance of a range of options are key, if clear and consistent messages are not being reinforced across all aspects of young people's lives – from the classroom, to the community, to health facilities, media outlets and within the home – young people are less likely to respond appropriately (Christopher, 1995; Franklin and Corcoran, 2000; Kirby, 2002bc).

So, the research evidence, from both poorer and richer countries, points to no 'harm' being done by sex and relationships education; indeed, the balance of the evidence points strongly to the protective effects of such programming.

Modes of delivery of sex and relationships programmes to young people

Across the world there are countless examples of programmes established in attempts to improve young people's knowledge, attitudes, skills and behaviours, some reporting greater success in their endeavours than others.

Programmes vary with respect to their content, aims, scope and method of implementation and delivery; however, what is clear is that taking a single strategy or message will not have the desired impact on every young person it reaches. The improvement of young people's sexual health through sex and relationships programming does not come in a 'one-size fits all' approach; what may work for a particular group of young people in a certain country context may fail miserably if used with another group. To guarantee as wide an impact as possible, the aim, therefore, is to provide a multifaceted, multi-sectoral, appropriate and cohesive response.

Programme settings

Although the range and content of sex and relationships programmes for young people is great, they can typically be organised according to four main programme settings: schools, mass media, communities, and the workplace or other non-formal educational settings. It is far beyond the scope of this chapter to provide a comprehensive review of all such approaches; indeed, this would fill a book by itself. Instead, the aim here is to briefly mention a range of such programmes and highlight some of the principles, opportunities, barriers and difficulties which are common to many, if not to all.

School-based educational programmes

Delivered primarily by teachers and typically based on a fixed curriculum, school-based educational programmes vary widely in content, delivery style and quality. Despite many problems including, among other things, lack of teacher training, time for, and timing of, delivery and limited consultation, such programmes have the potential to reach many young people in countries where school attendance is high and where its provision is official policy (for more, see Smith *et al.*, 2000; Family Health International, 2002).

Different countries use different names to cover their inputs; among these are *sexual and reproductive health education, family life education, personal development, life-skills education* or simply *sex education*. Although each aims to provide young people with accurate and comprehensive information to enable them to form attitudes and beliefs about sex, sexual identity and relationships, the emphases can vary markedly. For example, calling a course *family life education* implies that it is primarily preparing young people for married life and may have an emphasis on reproductive – as opposed to sexual – health issues. While these are certainly important, the coverage may be somewhat less comprehensive than a course entitled *sex and relationships* education. Similarly, courses that stress the importance of *life skills* may be based on the assumption that simply improving the social skills of young people will be sufficient to make a difference; they may, however, ignore the important issues relating to gender power relations, the effects of poverty, and so on (see Boler and Aggleton, 2005). In some cases, the designers of the course have a genuine belief that their approach is needed; in other cases, the selection of a name may be based on a pragmatic decision in the light of what would be acceptable to communities and families in particular countries.

Mass media

With their ability to reach large numbers of individuals with basic messages and information, the mass media (including radio, television, Internet, newspapers, magazines, billboards and direct mail-outs) have increasingly been utilised for the promotion of sexual health among young people. Although there is currently little evidence to suggest such techniques are directly influential on behaviour, they can be key strategies for the dissemination of knowledge and the development of social norms particularly among the so-called 'hard to reach' groups, including those not in school and those who have low literacy levels (FOCUS on Young Adults, 1997; Family Health International, 2002). Media coverage may also provide an opportunity for children and their parents to discuss issues when they are raised, for example, in a radio or television soap opera. Chapter 10 in this volume explores the potential role of the media in more detail.

Community-based programmes

Ranging from small-scale awareness-raising all the way through to community mobilisation efforts, such programmes and schemes are designed to address some of the powerful external influences that impact upon young people's lives. Although not always explicitly designed to include a sexual health component (and so diffusing potential conflict from conservative factions), many community based programmes can indirectly affect young people's sexual lives for the better (see Box 11.1 for example).

Non-formal setting based programmes

Many young people across the world miss out on the opportunity of a school-based education for a multitude of reasons including poverty, civil war, discrimination and displacement. Non-formal sex and relationships programmes, delivered from a variety of settings including young people's places of work and social arenas, are therefore an important way of reaching young people who might otherwise be overlooked. Delivered by either trained professionals or peers, such programmes can be an invaluable tool in reaching potentially higher risk young people (for some examples, see Safe Passages to Adulthood, 2002a, 2002b, 2002c).

Box 11.1

Young women in poverty are especially vulnerable to sexual ill-health not only due to lack of income, but also through lack of control of their lives. Often employed in jobs which attract low remuneration and long hours, young women are at increased risk of exploitation by employers in relation to receipt of gifts or favours in exchange for sex. Improving young women's financial status can enable them to take greater power over their lives and help them resist exploitation.

In Kenya, the Tap and Reposition Youth (TRY) savings and credit scheme, supported by K-REP Development Agency and Population Council, was established for out of school young women aged between 16 and 24 years living in low income and slum areas of Nairobi. The scheme, based on an existing credit, savings and business skills programme, provided basic training in business management to young women, including record keeping, marketing, pricing and customer relations. In addition, life skills and reproductive health issues such as family planning and HIV/AIDS awareness are addressed during sessions.

(Adapted from www.popcouncil.org/projects/TA_KenyaTRY.html).

Programme design/models

The pedagogic approach often adopted in sex and relationships education programmes draws on a number of psychologically-based behaviour and behavioural change theories that derive from a rationalist framework; these assume that a combination of one or more of appropriate information, attitudes, fear, perceived susceptibility, perceived vulnerability, and other variables, will lead to the development of intention to adopt safer behaviours. As has been demonstrated elsewhere in this volume, however, such simplistic models can not be directly applied to young people's sexual lives, which are strongly shaped and influenced by the resources available, longstanding cultural traditions and beliefs and the environment in which they are living. Programme designers therefore need to consider a much broader range of issues if a positive impact is to be achieved. Key among these are the issues of the social contexts and meanings of sexual activity.

By pointing to the limitations of these rational models, we need to stress that we are not implying that young people behave in an irrational way. Rather, we need to consider that there are a range of rationalities that influence young people, and that these need to be borne in mind in designing programmes (see Ingham *et al.*, 1992; Ingham, 1994). As an example, consider the pioneering work of Gagnon and Simon, who argued that young people, like adults, are limited by a specific set of 'cultural scripts' (both gender and non-gender based) which regulate their sex and sexuality, at the cultural, the interpersonal and the intra-psychic levels (Gagnon and

Simon, 1974; Simon and Gagnon, 1986; Gagnon and Parker, 1995; Hynie *et al.*, 1998).

For example, the negotiation of safer sexual practices through the use of condoms challenges culturally constructed notions (the 'scripts') of femininity and masculinity. All over the world, dominant ideologies of femininity work to bring about the passivity and submissiveness of women during sexual encounters, ideologies that are in conflict with the approaches that ask these same young women to act in non-conformist ways and become proactive to ensure the use of condoms during these encounters. Conversely, young men are expected to demonstrate their masculinity and dominance to safeguard their social and sexual reputations through showing sexual prowess and engaging in risk-taking activities (Waldby *et al.*, 1993; Lever, 1995; Holland *et al.*, 1998; Gavey *et al.*, 2001; Marston, 2004). In other words, the rationality of maintaining reputations dominates the rationality offered by the health promotion discourse. Similarly, earning money or gifts through sexual favours when living in extreme poverty can be seen as a perfectly rational way of behaving.

What to include in sex and relationships programmes for young people

Curriculum content

The potential content and scope of sex and relationships programmes is immense, and can encompass a vast range of issues. Priorities will vary from setting to setting according to the local priorities, but a good curriculum would typically cover three main areas; facts and information, relationships and interpersonal skills and values.

Facts and information

At the advent of sex and relationships programming, teachings mainly consisted of human biology, reproduction, hygiene and marriage. Although these still continue to be the main drivers in some parts of the world today (Smith *et al.*, 2000), many programmes have expanded to include the provision of accurate information on the physical and emotional changes associated with growing up, reproduction and sexually transmitted infections including HIV/AIDS. Furthermore, comprehensive curricula also cover contraception including the range of methods, how they work, how they can be obtained (together with any legal restrictions and issues of confidentiality), sources of advice and support, contraceptive decision-making, abortion and sexual abuse.

Relationships and interpersonal skills

Well-designed sex and relationships programmes should seek to provide young people with the opportunity to consider relationship diversity, marriage and partnership, love and commitment and the law relating to sexual behaviour and relationships, as well as the range of religious, societal and cultural views on sex, sexuality and sexual diversity. They should also encourage young people to challenge and question social stereotypes, tackle issues of gender and power and develop a range of other skills, including communication, negotiation, decision-making, critical thinking, assertiveness and refusal skills, to assist them in their sexual lives.

Values

One of the criticisms levelled at some comprehensive approaches to sex and relationships education is that it is value-free; it is argued that the only way that such issues can and should be covered is within a clear moral framework that stresses the centrality of sex occurring within the context of heterosexual marriage. For those young people who have aligned with a particular religious or cultural value-system, such approaches may be helpful. However, for the majority of young people in many parts of the world this approach is simply irrelevant and hopelessly idealistic. Further, it is a mistake to believe that other approaches are value-free; for example, approaches that stress the crucial importance of the values of mutuality and respect – for oneself and for others – should lead to delay or self-restraint until such a time as individuals feel both physically and emotionally ready to engage in sexual relations free from social pressures, and should also lead to increased use of protection, and recognition of the right of every individual to sexual fulfilment free from coercion and stigma.

A further criticism made by opponents of comprehensive approaches to sex and relationships education, especially in school settings, is that they undermine the role of the family in bringing up their children. The reality is that the extent of discussion between parents and their children on sexual matters is generally minimal. What is important to develop is good communication between schools (and other agencies) and parents (subject to the respect for confidentiality) so that each party knows what the others are doing; in this way, young people should avoid receiving mixed and confusing messages, and the relative contribution of schools and families – in terms of knowledge, skills and values – can be agreed. Indeed, programme planners could do more to encourage discussion within families and to support parents who wish to offer more protection to their children but who feel ill-equipped to do so.

Modes of delivery

Many school-based programmes continue to rely on didactic forms of delivery of sex and relationships education issues, in line with other aspects of the curricula. Although such an approach might be more appropriate for some of the more factual aspects of the curriculum, it is not at all suitable for the skills and values aspects. Small group, more participatory approaches are strongly recommended, in which young people are encouraged to: discuss situations and develop their own 'solutions'; work out their own value systems; practice, through role-playing and other methods, how to deal with specific situations; and so on. The use of well-prepared peers in these endeavours has been strongly recommended (UNAIDS, 1999).

Abstinence-only approaches

The growth of the abstinence-only approach to sex and relationships education in recent years warrants special attention. No one could argue with the proposition that abstaining from any form of sexual contact (both inside and outside of marriage) is the most effective way of preventing the transmission of STIs and HIV/AIDS. However, not only do such programmes abuse the rights of young people (as outlined earlier), there is little evidence that they are at all effective in achieving their aims. Their increasing spread in the USA and some other countries is being matched by attempts to impose them on poorer countries through restrictions placed on the USA's overseas development programme.

Internationally, financial support for abstinence-based sex and relationships programmes has never been so great. For instance, in 2003, the US Congress passed legislation that authorised up to $15 billion over five years to implement their President's Emergency Plan for AIDS Relief (PEPFAR) in response to the AIDS pandemic in targeted sub-Saharan and Caribbean nations (Office of the Press Secretary, 2003, 2004). Authorised programme activities included stressing the gains to be realised through abstaining from sexual activity until marriage, and restricting condom promotion to those who cannot avoid high-risk behaviours. The Act states that a third of all monies authorised for prevention purposes must be used for services that promote abstinence-until-marriage (Library of Congress, 2003). Further, funding is only granted to local organisations that have a 'policy explicitly opposing prostitution and sex trafficking' (see, for example, CDC, 2005).

The research evidence on which the abstinence-only approach is based is flimsy, to say the least. Two key evaluation methods have been used, both using data from the USA; one evaluated the impact of school-based programmes and the other followed up a cohort of young people who had voluntarily signed the 'virginity pledge'.

Kirby's careful assessment of the effect of school-based programmes led him to conclude that:

> ... the evidence is not conclusive about the impact of abstinence-only programs ... there do not currently exist any abstinence-only programs

with reasonably strong evidence that they actually delay the initiation of sex or reduce its frequency ... [but] one should not conclude that all abstinence-only programs either do or do not delay sex.

(Kirby, 2001: 6)

More recently, Santelli *et al.* (2006: 79), after reviewing a number of previous reviews and other material, conclude that 'abstinence-only programs are inconsistent with commonly accepted notions of human rights' and that '"Abstinence-only" as a basis for health policy and programs should be abandoned'.

The cohort studies use data from the large Adolescent Health Surveys that have been conducted in the USA over the past few years; using data from three waves of an original sample of over 12,000 young people, researchers have been able to track the fate of those who reported having signed up to a virginity pledge during their early teenage years (Bearman and Brückner, 2001, 2004; Brückner and Bearman, 2005). By wave two of the study, they identified the characteristics of those who had signed up to the pledge; these included being more religious, being bodily less mature, being less cognitively able, and having more 'normative values' on romantic love and gender relations. The authors report that pledgers, when compared with non-pledgers, did show a delay in their first intercourse, but that contraceptive use was about one-third lower when they did have sex for the first time.

By wave three of the study, some six years after the start, a very high proportion of pledgers reported sexual activity. Again, condom use was lower among the failed pledgers. The study included testing for sexually transmitted infections and found that the rate among the failed pledgers was not significantly different from that found for the non-pledgers. Indeed, in communities where the proportion of pledgers had been higher than 20 per cent, the rates of STIs were almost twice as high as in communities with lower proportions. The authors propose that failing pledgers in the higher pledging communities are at higher risk of STIs, since they need to keep their sexual activity more hidden (to avoid the embarrassment of admitting to having 'failed') and so are less likely to have been previously tested for STIs. Other researchers have reported similar outcomes for the impact of pledging virginity until marriage (for example, Jemmott *et al.*, 1998; Lipsitz *et al.*, 2003; Henry J Kaiser Family Foundation, 2003).

That a large number of those young people who choose to try to remain 'virgins' until marriage not only fail in their efforts but also, under some conditions, have poorer physical sexual health (and possibly more feelings of shame and guilt), does not augur well for the impact of compulsory abstinence-only programmes. These results indicate that the imposition of this particular moralistically based approach serves not only to deny young people their rights to the full range of risk-reduction options, but also puts them at higher risk of negative sexual health outcomes. We do, of course, need to be clear regarding the difference between *abstinence-only* approaches, with their emphasis on waiting until marriage and on the unreliability of contraception, and approaches that stress the desirability of *delaying* early sex until such time as people choose to do what they wish with whom they wish, free from coercion from partners or peers.

Conclusions

Throughout the world, both adults and young people alike have begun to reconsider their beliefs and values concerning appropriate sexual behaviour in response to increasing rates of unintended pregnancy, and fears of STIs and HIV/AIDS. However, the provision of information alone will not achieve the desired level of behaviour change and adoption of safer-sex practices necessary among young people. Significant barriers to change continue to exist in many countries, frequently a reflection of the political, legal, economic, social and cultural contexts of the environment in which young people live. For instance, advising young people about the need to protect themselves from unwanted pregnancy, STIs and HIV through the use of condoms is futile if they are unable to obtain them, because of insufficient funds, lack of service provision or even legal restrictions. Once condoms have been obtained, their correct use has to be communicated and negotiated with partners which can require great confidence and skill, particularly for young women if partners are spouses, dominant or aggressive, or possibly unknown. Further, negative social connotations of protected sex may dominate.

With increased globalisation young people's knowledge and attitudes to sex and sexuality are constructed and shaped at a variety of levels and from a range of sources including each other, kinship networks, community and wider-society, religion, media, and so on. Similarly, young people's sexual health information resources are numerous and diverse with some of the information received being accurate and some less so. The key role, therefore, of sex and relationships programming is to ensure that young people's knowledge is complete, that misinformation and beliefs are dispelled, that suitable skills are developed and that appropriate culturally sensitive values are clarified, for without these foundations young people will remain vulnerable to negative sexual health outcomes.

References

AGI (2001) *Can More Progress be Made? Teenage Sexual and Reproductive Behavior in Developed Countries,* New York: The Alan Guttmacher Institute.

Bearman, P. and Brückner, H. (2001) Promising the future: Virginity pledges and first intercourse, *American Journal of Sociology,* 106(4), 859–912.

Bearman, P. and Brückner, H. (2004) *The Relationship between Virginity Pledges in Adolescence and STD Acquisition in Young Adulthood,* paper presented at the National STD Conference, 9 March 2004, Philadelphia, PA.

Boler, T. and Aggleton, P. (2005) *Life Skills-based Education for HIV Prevention: A critical analysis,* Policy and Research, issue 3. London: Save the Children and ActionAid International.

Bozon, M. and Kontula, O. (1998) Sexual initiation and gender: A cross-cultural analysis of trends in the 20th century, in Hubert, M., Bajos, N. and Sandfort, Th. (eds) *Sexual Behaviour and Trends in Europe: Comparisons of national surveys,* London: UCL Press, 181–93.

Brown, A.D., Jeejebhoy, S.J., Shah, I. and Yount, K.M. (2001) *Sexual Relations Among Young People in Developing Countries: Evidence from WHO case studies,* Geneva: World Health Organistion.

Brückner, H. and Bearman, P. (2005) After the promise: The STD consequences of adolescent virginity pledges, *Journal of Adolescent Health,* 36, 271–78.

CDC (Centers for Disease Control) (2005) *Increasing Access to HIV Counseling and Testing and Enhancing HIV/AIDS Communications, Prevention and Care in Botswana, Lesotho, South Africa, Swaziland and Côte d'Ivoire,* billing code 4163–18-P, Atlanta GA: Department of Health and Human Services, CDC (available at <www.cdc.gov/od/pgo/funding/AA006.htm>).

Christopher, F.S. (1995) Adolescent pregnancy prevention, *Family Relations,* 44(4), 384–91.

Family Health International (2002) *Intervention Strategies that Work for Youth: Summary of FOCUS on young adults end of programme report,* Arlington, VA: Family Health International.

FOCUS on Young Adults (1997) *Promoting Reproductive Health for Young Adults through Social Marketing and Mass Media: A review of trends and practices,* Washington DC: FOCUS on Young Adults.

Franklin, C. and Corcoran, J. (2000) Preventing adolescent pregnancy: A review of programs and practices, *Social Work,* 45(1), 40–52.

Franklin, C., Grant D., Corcoran, J., Miller, P.O. and Bultman, L. (1997) Effectiveness of prevention programs for adolescent pregnancy: A meta-analysis, *Journal of Marriage and the Family,* 59(3), 551–67.

Gagnon, J. and Simon, W. (1974) *Sexual Conduct: The social sources of human sexuality,* London: Hutchinson.

Gagnon, J. and Parker, G. (1995) Conceiving sexuality, in Parker, R. and Gagnon, J. (eds) *Conceiving Sexuality: Approaches to sex research in a post-modern world,* London: Routledge, 3–16.

Gavey, N., McPhillips, K. and Doherty, M. (2001) 'If it's not on, it's not on' – or is it? Discursive constraints on women's condom use, *Gender and Society,* 15(6), 917–34.

Grunseit, A., Kippax, S., Aggleton, P., Baldo, M. and Slutkin, G. (1997) Sexuality education and young people's sexual behavior: A review of studies, *Journal of Adolescent Research,* 12(4), 421–53.

Henry J. Kaiser Family Foundation (2003) *Seventeen: Virginity and the first time,* Menlo Park, CA: Kaiser Family Foundation.

Holland, J., Ramazanoglu, C., Sharpe, S. and Thomson, R. (1998) *The Male in the Head: Young people, heterosexuality and power,* London: Tufnell Press.

Hynie, M., Lydon, J., Cote, S. and Wiener, S. (1998) Relational sexual scripts and women's condom use: The importance of internalized norms, *Journal of Sex Research*, 35(4), 370–80.

Ingham, R. (1994) Some speculations on the concept of rationality, in G. Albrecht (ed.) *Advances in Medical Sociology, Vol. IV: A reconsideration of models of health behavior change*, Greenwich, CN, JAI Press, 89–111.

Ingham, R. (2005) We didn't cover that at school: Education against pleasure or education for pleasure? *Sex Education*, 5(4), 375–88.

Ingham, R., Woodcock, A. and Stenner, K. (1992) The limitations of rational decision making models as applied to young people's sexual behaviour, in Aggleton, P., Davies, P. and Hart, G. (eds) *AIDS: Rights, risk and reason*, London: Falmer Press, 163–73.

Jemmott, J., Jemmott, L. and Fong, G. (1998) Abstinence and safer sex HIV risk-reduction interventions for African American adolescents, *Journal of the American Medical Association*, 279(19), 1529–36.

Kirby, D. (1997) *No Easy Answers*, Washington, DC: National Campaign to Prevent Teen Pregnancy.

Kirby, D. (2001) *Emerging Answers: Research findings on programs to reduce teen pregnancy*, Washington, DC: National Campaign to Prevent Teen Pregnancy.

Kirby, D. (2002a) *Do Abstinence-only Programs Delay the Initiation of Sex among Young People and Reduce Teen Pregnancy?* Washington, DC: National Campaign to Prevent Teen Pregnancy.

Kirby, D. (2002b) The impact of schools and school programs upon adolescent sexual behavior, *Journal of Sex Research*, 39(1), 27–33.

Kirby, D. (2002c) Effective approaches to reducing adolescent unprotected sex, pregnancy, and childbearing, *Journal of Sex Research*, 39(1), 51–7.

Lever, J. (1995) Bringing the fundamentals of gender studies into safer-sex education, *Family Planning Perspectives*, 27(4), 172–74.

Library of Congress (2003) *To Provide Assistance to Foreign Countries to Combat HIV/AIDS, Tuberculosis and Malaria, and for Other Purposes*, H.R.1298, Public Law No, 108–25, house report 108–60, Washington DC: Library of Congress.

Lipsitz, A., Bishop, P. and Robinson, C. (2003) Virginity pledges: Who takes them and how well do they work? presentation at the Annual Convention of the American Psychological Association, Altanta, 29 May – 1 June.

Marston, C. (2004) Gendered communication among young people in Mexico: Implications for sexual health interventions, *Social Science and Medicine*, 59(3), 445–56.

McNab, W. (1981) Advocating elementary sex education, *Health Education*, 12, 22–5.

Office of the Press Secretary (2003) *Fact Sheet: The President's Emergency Plan for AIDS Relief*, Washington DC: The White House.

Office of the Press Secretary (2004) *Fact Sheet: Extending and Improving the Lives of Those Living with HIV/AIDS*, Washington DC: The White House.

Safe Passages to Adulthood (2002a) *Working with Young Men to Promote Sexual and Reproductive Health*, Southampton: University of Southampton, Centre for Sexual Health Research, Safe Passages to Adulthood programme.

Safe Passages to Adulthood (2002b) *The Role of Education in Promoting Young People's Sexual and Reproductive Health*, Southampton: University of

Southampton, Centre for Sexual Health Research, Safe Passages to Adulthood programme.

Safe Passages to Adulthood and WHO (2002c) *Preventing HIV/AIDS and Promoting Sexual Health among Especially Vulnerable Young People,* Southampton: University of Southampton, Centre for Sexual Health Research, Safe Passages to Adulthood programme.

Santelli, J., Ott, M.A., Lyon, M., Rogers, J., Summers, D. and Schleifer, R. (2006) Abstinence and abstinence-only education: A review of US policies and programs, *Journal of Adolescent Health,* 38, 72–81.

Simon, W. and Gagnon, J. (1986) Sexual scripts: Permanence and change, *Archives of Sexual Behavior,* 15(2), 97–120.

Smith, G., Kippax, S. and Aggleton, P. (2000) *HIV and Sexual Health Education in Primary and Secondary Schools: Findings from selected Asia-Pacific countries,* Sydney: The University of New South Wales, National Centre in HIV Social Research.

UN (1989) *UN Convention on the Rights of the Child,* Geneva: UN High Commission for Human Rights.

UN (1993) *Declaration on the Elimination of Violence against Women,* Geneva: UN High Commission for Human Rights.

UN (1994) *Population and Development, Vol. 1: Programme of action adopted at the international conference on population and development,* (ICPD), Cairo, 5 –13 September. New York: Department of Economic and Social Information and Policy Analysis, United Nations.

UN (1999) *Key Actions of the Further Implementation of the Programme of Action of the International Conference on Population and Development,* (A/S-21/5/Add.1) (ICPD+5), New York: United Nations.

UNAIDS (1997) *Impact of HIV and Sexual Health Education on the Sexual Behaviour of Young People: A review update,* Geneva: Switzerland, UNAIDS.

UNAIDS (1999) Peer education and HIV/AIDS: Concepts, uses and challenges, Geneva: UNAIDS (UNAIDS/99.46E).

UNAIDS (2004) *2004 Report on the Global* AIDS *Epidemic,* Geneva: UNAIDS.

UNICEF (2001) *A League Table of Teenage Births in Rich Nations,* Innocenti Report Card 3, Florence: UNICEF.

Waldby, C., Kippax, S. and Crawford, J. (1993) Research Note – Heterosexual men and safe sex practice, *Sociology of Health and Illness,* 15(2), 46–56.

Chapter 12

Research and policy in young people's sexual health[1]

Roger Ingham and Susannah Mayhew

Introduction

This chapter considers the links between research and the policy process, and the particular challenges faced in the field of young people's sexual and reproductive health. We consider the key players and their relationships, discuss some important dynamics that need to be considered in attempting to effect change, and explore some practical issues concerning communication and influence. Some of the personalities and politics that influence the research-policy interface in the field of young people's sexual health are illustrated by examples drawn from current debates in the field, particularly on abstinence and HIV/AIDS.

Policy development from formulation to implementation, and the influence of research on this process, is highly complex. The processes involved are non-linear and often appear irrational since they are influenced by a diverse range of players, by the particularities of the political process and by the social context (Walt, 1994; Trostle *et al.*, 1999; Black, 2001; Nolan, 2002). It must be stressed at the outset that the chapter cannot provide a blueprint for successful action; rather, it aims to consider just a few of the issues that need to be taken into account. Neither is it an academic review of the more formal theories that have been developed in this area; for such analyses, the reader is directed to Walt (1994) and Buse *et al.* (2005). As will be shown, the area of sexual and reproductive health is especially complex compared with other areas of health because of the fine line between public and private action and the sensitivity and controversy surrounding sexuality and its consequences. For example, there is almost certainly widespread agreement that reducing rates of child deaths from malaria or diarrhoea would be beneficial. In such cases, the flow from research on a solution to policy development and implementation of that solution may be fairly straightforward (in theory, at least), with the main barriers being technical and financial.

The field of sexual and reproductive health, however, poses considerable additional challenges that need to be considered; these include a whole raft of religious, cultural, social and community attitudes that affect the responses of those in positions of influence. The history of family planning research and interventions is replete with examples of how seemingly well-meaning approaches have foundered when confronted with some of these barriers (see, for example, the edited collection by Russell *et al.*, 2000); the intentions of researchers, donors, advocacy groups and policy-makers have been questioned, mutual suspicions have arisen and forms of resistance have developed.

Adding 'young people', 'youth' or 'adolescents' into the field raises additional challenges. Although there may be general agreement that early and unplanned pregnancy, high rates of STIs and HIV, and abortion-related complications and deaths should be reduced, quite how, and at what cost, these outcomes should be achieved is a matter of intense disagreement. For example, some religious organisations might never countenance certain changes no matter how powerful is the research evidence against their particular views; the refusal of the Catholic church to officially promote the use of condoms is a prime example, as is the dissemination of the view that condoms have 'holes' in them (BBC, 2003). Similarly, there is a widespread view in many cultures that informing young people about sexual health issues will encourage them to become sexually active at a stage when this is not felt to be appropriate (that is, in many cases, before they are married to someone of the opposite sex). Given the very close relations in some countries between political and religious organisations, these factors can profoundly influence the relationship between research and policy.

Policy-makers are under increasing pressure to show that their policies are 'evidence-based' or 'evidence-informed'. The opportunity for researchers to influence policy therefore is perhaps greater than it has ever been. In reality, policy-makers may use, manipulate or ignore research. Understanding the drivers of policy and the pathways and actions through which research can successfully engage with the policy process is highly complex. The following discussions of the key players, strategies and approaches and how these are affected by personalities and politics, is an attempt to shed light on the important interface between these two realms of practice.

Key players and their relationships

We start by outlining who the key players are in the whole dynamic process through which policies become formulated, altered and implemented. There are four main groups of players, although there can be overlap between categories: policy-makers, researchers, funders and donors, and mediators. First, the policy-makers are those who, through election, appointment, invitation, choice or other routes, are in positions to make decisions that affect aspects of what is, or should be, carried out in the field. We can, to some extent, distinguish between what might be called '*BIG P*' from what we will call 'little p'. The 'BIG P' tend to be politicians or decision-makers working in national government structures and bi/multilateral agencies. These players are concerned with international or national laws, policies, strategies, and guidelines that affect some aspect of sexual and reproductive health, be this through education, health systems, public campaigns, laws, stigma and discrimination, and a wide range of other issues. Policy-makers with a 'little p' are the decision-makers who are more concerned with the implementation of approaches in sub-national institutions and everyday situations; thus, for example, a school teacher can be regarded as a policy-maker or decision-taker to the extent that he or she decides what should be covered in (or omitted from) lessons within a sex and relationships education curriculum. The individual teacher will, in most cases, be influenced by others – their head teacher, the school's governors (or equivalent), the views of parents, views in the local community, and others. Similarly, a health worker in a sexual health clinic will implement the policy of that clinic in terms of who they see, their attitude towards the 'client', their reactions to issues of confidentiality and so on. Even in cases where services and educational establishments have clear policies in place, individual interpretations of what is expected of the staff may vary considerably, as might the level of sanctions imposed by management on staff who breach the policy guidelines. To further add to the complexity, policy implementation in a school may be undermined by parents or carers who happen to take a different view; in this sense, everyone has a domain of influence that can affect the development or implementation of policy.

There is not necessarily any relationship between 'BIG P' and 'little p' aspects of the policy process. In some places, there are good national policies in place regarding young people and sexual health, but little evidence on the ground that these are either known about or being implemented. In other places, there may be good local practice but no national policies. In yet others, there may be clear national policies that are actively opposed by those on the ground because they do not agree with them. As an example, consider the case of the UN Convention on the Rights of the Child. One hundred and forty countries in the world have signed up to this of which all but two have ratified the Convention. Signatories are expected periodically to report to the UN system what progress they have made towards the objectives. And yet is it abundantly clear that the expectations and obligations contained within the Convention are largely ignored in some places (see Box 12.1).

Box 12.1 Abstinence-only policies violate the Convention on the Rights of the Child (CRC) (UN, 1989)

The USA is one of two countries that have signed the CRC but failed to ratify it – that is to make good their intentions at a domestic level by enacting/amending laws to support the aims of the Convention. Nevertheless, the fact that it has signed means the USA remains under an obligation to *refrain, from acts that would defeat the object and the purpose of the treaty* (Article 18, Vienna Convention on the Law of Treaties, 1969, (see www. untreaty.un.org/law/ilc/texts/instruments/english/conventions/l_l_1969.pdf).

The Convention on the Rights of the Child is explicit in safeguarding the child's right to information: *The child shall have the right to freedom of expression; this right shall include freedom to seek, receive and impart information and ideas of all kinds* (UN, 1989: Article 13.1).

The practical realities of this are laid out in the CRC's General Comment 3 on HIV/AIDS and General Comment 4 (UN, 2003ab) on Adolescent Health: ... *effective HIV/AIDS prevention requires States to refrain from censoring, withholding or intentionally misrepresenting health-related information including sexual education and information* (CRC/GC/2003/3: para. 16) *and It is the obligation of States parties to ensure that all adolescent girls and boys both in and out of school, are provided with and not denied, accurate and appropriate information on how to protect their health ...* (CRC/GC/2003/4: para. 26).

Recognising that adolescents are at risk of being infected with STDs including HIV/AIDS, the CRC states that: *States parties are urged ... to take measures to remove all barriers hindering the access of adolescents to information, preventive measures such as condoms and care.* (CRC/GC/2003/4: para. 30).

As a signatory to the CRC, the USA is bound not to maintain or enact laws that are counter to the above obligations, and yet the abstinence-only policy being widely implemented across schools in the US southern states is in explicit violation of these obligations.

A report (the Waxman Report) for the US House of Representatives in 2004 stated that ... *over 80 per cent of abstinence-only curricula ... contain false, misleading, or distorted information about reproductive health* (US House of Representatives, 2004: i).

Human Rights Watch investigated the impact of this abstinence-only policy on what was being taught in schools and concluded that such policies: ... *systematically deny children basic information that could protect them from HIV/AIDS infection ... these programs interfere with fundamental rights to information, to health and to equal protection under the law. They also place children at unnecessary risk of HIV infection and premature death* (Human Rights Watch, 2002: 46). Interviews conducted for this study indicate the severity of the impact of the policy: *We don't talk about HIV/AIDS prevention ... we don't mention the word 'condoms' at all.* Headmaster, Texas (Human Rights Watch 2002: 19) and *I don't know any other way but abstinence to prevent HIV.* Schoolgirl, 16, Texas (Human Rights Watch, 2002: 20).

The impact of US policies is also making itself felt through conditions attached to their assistance to African countries most affected by HIV/AIDS. Uganda has both signed and ratified the CRC, and yet a Ugandan schoolteacher relates that since US funding increased: *We were told not to show [pupils] how to use condoms and not to talk about them at our school. In the past we used to show them ... Now we can't do that* (Human Rights Watch, 2005: 34).

The second group of players are *researchers*. These may operate from academic establishments or from private and/or charitable organisations, and may receive funding from governments, charities, private donors, or elsewhere (Peterson, 2002). Their research may be self-generated and/or commissioned by one or more of the sources of finance. The source of funding may influence the design of the research and the interpretation of results (Rampton and Stauber, 2001). The researchers themselves may carry out the research from a completely neutral stance or they may have pre-conceived ideas of what they hope to find, particularly if they are influenced by their funding source (McKee *et al.*, 2001 (chapter 8); Collin *et al.*, 2002). Their main audiences will vary, with some being primarily concerned with influencing policy-makers in a direct way, while others may be more motivated by their own academic advancement and chances of promotion (some will fluctuate between these motivations, others will attempt to achieve both, and so on). Some research will be primarily theory-driven and some will have more practical and even pragmatic aims, such as operations research, needs assessments, audits, and process and outcome evaluations.

The third set of key players in the relationship are the *funders* and *donors*. Varying considerably in size and aims, where they choose to focus their attention and their money has a major impact on which areas are prioritised for policy attention as well as which research areas are funded. Some large funders are, of course, linked with governments (for example, USAID and DFID) while others are independent, such as the Ford, Packard and Gates Foundations. The former group fund research that will be supportive of, and restricted by, their national policy directions, while the latter group generally have freedom from such constraints. Other research funders (research councils, for example) receive government money but maintain academic independence (in theory, at least) to fund work as they choose. Peer review of research submissions may be purely by other academics, or may include the more active involvement of policy-makers who evaluate the likely impact of the results on practical implementation.

Finally, a rather fluid but important group comprises what might be termed the *intermediaries* or *mediators*. As the name suggests, these organisations or individuals act as go-betweens, linking policy-makers with researchers, both intentionally and unintentionally, in a range of manners. Mediators may include think-tanks (such as the Overseas Development Institute, or the Fabian Society in the UK) who commission research and use the results to develop policy which is then proposed to national governments and other agencies. Some (for example, interest groups or non-governmental organisations like Human Rights Watch or Catholics for Free Choice) have more explicit international or national advocacy functions, and promote research evidence that can be used to support their particular focus. Local interest groups operate in local settings and make links with communities and key agencies to encourage communication and understanding around a policy issue. In many ways the media also act as brokers or mediators; for example, the press can take up (and whip up) popular opinion based on real or erroneously-interpreted research that puts pressure on the Government to act to change policy (Miller, 1999; Cole *et al.*, 2002).

'Evidence', values and motivation

A critical set of issues emerging from the above discussion concerns the construction of 'evidence' and the particular values and motivations of the different stakeholders.

Constructing 'evidence'

In theory at least, research is supposed to be value-free, whereas policy priorities are normally located within a wider political, ideological or moral framework (Russell *et al.*, 2000; Nolan, 2002). In reality, research can be subjectively created, selected and interpreted (Black, 2001). As noted earlier, research can be influenced by who funds and who 'owns' it. Political forces and views can also shape which evidence is selected to shape policy and opinions (Brickman *et al.*, 1985). The stance of South African President Thabo Mbeki on AIDS is a classic example. His now infamous position to the effect that a virus cannot cause a syndrome, that a virus can cause a disease and that AIDS is not a disease but a syndrome, was backed up with a body of scientific research 'evidence', albeit long rejected by mainstream Western scientists. Mbeki as a black President of South Africa selected his evidence to mount a challenge to Western orthodoxy and dominance to the point of dismissing 'Western' bio-medical research. Scientific research became a weapon in the political 'battle between certain state and non-state actors to define who has the right to speak about AIDS, to determine the response to AIDS and even to define the problem itself' (Schneider, 2002: 153).

Policy-makers may also selectively, or uncritically, interpret evidence when they feel under pressure to produce positive outcomes. The early official Ugandan interpretation of their AIDS 'decline', for example, which was heralded as Africa's big success story, was in fact based on a very few pieces of selective 'evidence' (Parkhurst, 2002).

Why is research commissioned?

Among the positive reasons for commissioning research are a genuine desire on the part of the policy-makers to improve matters in relation to young people's sexual and reproductive health, to help to develop long-term strategies, to explore the costs and benefits of particular courses of action, to assist in developing a stronger case for investing in young people's services and education, to explore more efficient means by which stigma and discrimination might be overcome, to collect the views of those affected by potential policies so that change is genuinely participatory, and so on. In other cases, however, there may be other – less positive – motivations at work. Such a list might include, for example, commissioning research as a device to postpone a decision when under pressure to act, to strengthen the position of civil servants over politicians, to placate international donors and others, to explore the cheapest option that will be acceptable, and so on.

Why do researchers do sexual health research?

Similarly, there is a range of reasons why researchers become involved in sexual health research; indeed, most will have multiple reasons. Some, operating from a 'pure' and objective position, have a genuine wish better to understand the enigmatic nature of sexual activity, to develop improved theories, to test innovative methodologies, to explore sexual health issues alongside other aspects of young people's development, and so on. Others may operate at the level of 'BIG P', and be motivated by a genuine desire to enhance young people's health and rights through macro-policy or programme changes, for example, to improve facilities and education for young people, either in general, or in relation to some particular aspect, such as gender relations, sexual diversity, violence and abuse; to help to develop a supportive and enabling environment for young people; to discourage early school-leaving among young women; and so on. Others will be more focused on 'little p' matters, such as improving staff attitudes in health services, to identify specific cultural and community barriers to change, to find better ways of evaluating effectiveness of programmes, to improve training of teachers and health service staff, to explore alternative modes of delivery in school settings, and so on.

Cutting across all of these motivations is a set of values regarding young people in general and sexual issues in particular; many researchers operate from a position of wishing to improve the choices available to young people within a liberal-humanist framework. Others, however, may disagree with young people having any sexual relations at all, and are motivated by a wish to find new ways of encouraging abstinence and delay. The choice of issue to be researched in the first place is often determined by the general value-system held by the researchers involved, and the line between research and advocacy can sometimes appear to be rather flimsy.

Strategic decisions

In many countries, there is a strong reluctance to discuss sexual matters, especially those involving young and unmarried people, those whose sexual preferences are towards their own sex, those who adopt lifestyles that may be illegal or strongly sanctioned, and so on. Many in positions of influence may rather ignore the area than have to deal with such troublesome issues. In other words, no matter how important a piece of research is, or how well-conducted the research may be, or how clearly the results point in a particular policy direction, there will still be barriers to be overcome if the work is to be funded and the results accepted. In addition to the widespread reluctance to accept and openly discuss young people's sexuality, there will be objections to some research results on ideological and/or religious grounds.

Given these sensitivities surrounding young people's sexual and repro-ductive health, it is particularly important to have a clear strategy or range of strategies in place to increase the probability of acceptance of research and its findings in this area. We know that research is more likely to influ-ence policy and practice if it is timely, topical, well-funded and engages early on with the interests and needs of policy-makers (Davis and Howden-Chapman, 1996). These and other key strategic factors are discussed below.

Factors influencing the policy-research interface

Timescales

Generally, policy-makers and decision-takers want relatively fast answers to a problem that is seen as urgent, whereas researchers tend to take rather longer to arrive at their results (and often end their papers with calls for fur-ther research before clear conclusions can be drawn). Greater communication between policy-makers and researchers on the aims of research could help researchers to appreciate the need to make short-term or 'interim' recommendations and policy-makers to acknowledge the value of longer-term research.

Approaches and clarity

Many researchers are concerned with theoretical and/or methodological development, whereas many policy-makers are often more pragmatic in their approach. Policy-makers need clear guidance on what they should do, and prefer simple solutions to act upon. Researchers are prone to being rather more circumspect in their conclusions, emphasising the complexity of situations. Again, closer consultation could achieve mutual recognition of the need for both simple short-term and more complex, longer-term rec-ommendations.

Language and assumptions

The demands of the more academic researchers for clear operational and the-oretical definitions and distinctions sometimes conflict with a rather simpler view of the world held by some policy-makers. Establishing formal communication channels and elimination by researchers of unnecessary use of jargon can enhance policy-research interaction.

Disciplinary divisions and policy requirements

Many researchers work within a specific disciplinary context, but the policy and programmatic challenges posed by HIV and other threats to sexual health require a multidisciplinary approach. This may mean forging new partnerships among researchers to ensure that as many aspects as possible are considered. This can create tensions, especially when researchers are evaluated within their own disciplinary boundaries for promotion, research assessment exercises, and other processes, but also has many advantages.

Capacity constraints and lack of political will

A set of recommendations made by researchers to address a particular issue may be ignored or overruled due to financial or other constraints, leading to frustration and resentment on the part of the research team that carried out the work and made the recommendations. Similarly, policy-makers may be reluctant to implement recommendations for fear of public reaction, loss of votes in forthcoming elections, loss of confidence among other stakeholders, because they want to 'own' the decision, or simply because they do not agree with the results. Again, researchers may feel aggrieved at having their work ignored. Closer and more formal interaction can help to manage expectations and minimise tension.

Engaging with policy- and decision-makers

Engaging with policy- and decision-makers and the policy process is critical if the policy-research divide is to be bridged. Researchers need to be aware of who the key decision makers are, including non-government groups who wield influence, and who will actually make the decisions. Researchers must then strive to achieve a consensus around values and convincingly present their case.

Striving for shared values and goals

A crucial component of increasing the chances of getting research results put into practice is that there are shared – or at least agreed – values and/or goals between the various parties involved. An initial stage of the process of influence will therefore need to be to persuade those in authority, and others with influence, that young people's sexual and reproductive health is indeed an issue to be addressed. As mentioned earlier, some people prefer to deny that young people engage in sexual activity at all, or that, if they do so, then they 'deserve' whatever fate befalls them. For example, some of the early WHO questionnaire surveys used in many countries in the late 1980s (Cleland and Ferry, 1995) omitted any items on masturbation and same-sex activities; the in-country planning teams often simply denied that any such activities occurred in their own countries. Similarly, some decision-makers in more 'traditional' countries may argue that young people do not engage in sex until they are married. So, prior to any efforts to implement the results of research into policy or practice, a process of sensitisation to issues is crucial.

This may involve some compromise on behalf of one or more of the agencies involved; for example, the speed of change that is expected by researchers and/or intermediaries may not be realistic in the context of specific cultural, political and financial contexts, so some phasing of goals may be required. What is crucial is that there is an agreed end-point, with mutual understanding of the necessary steps by which this can be achieved, both in the short-term and the medium- to longer-term (see Chapter 9 in this volume). Among these shared goals, there needs to be agreement on what will count as 'success' at various points along the path. Shared goals on young people and sexual health issues often include reduction of the rates of STIs including HIV, or the numbers of early unplanned pregnancies (and associated terminations).

The importance of networks and discussion fora

It is vital that the different parties involved maintain close contact during the process of initial decisions, commissioning, carrying out the research and deciding the most effective means of implementing the findings. In this way, possible misunderstandings and suspicions can be overcome, all involved can be reassured that they are working for a common agreed cause, and responsibility for processes and outcomes are shared. Each party needs to recognise the expertise of the others; while researchers may be the experts in designing and executing the research itself, the policy-makers should be the experts in knowing what is needed and what is feasible in terms of implementation. Issues such as the use of different languages or discourses, different ways of understanding the issues involved, and so on, can often be overcome during the planning meetings. Equally, where researchers run into practical problems in carrying out the research (which is often the case) then a well-networked advisory group, including political decision makers, can be immensely helpful in finding solutions and helping to solve the dilemmas.

A crucial part of any good research network and advisory group is the close involvement of the young people who may be the focus of the research. Before any questionnaire or qualitative tool is finalised, it is essential that the views of young people are obtained in order to ensure that the language is suitable, that the issues are clear, and that misunderstandings will be minimised. Such involvement may also assist researchers in gaining access to samples that may be difficult to reach through other means.

In arguing the case for research funding, and in publicising the results, many groups have found it extremely useful to have public meetings at which the relevant issues can be discussed openly and in some detail. Hearing young people speaking about the issues as they understand and experience them is valuable in persuading the decision-makers of their needs and rights, and also in alerting researchers to the issues that warrant their attention.

Presenting a case

Given the often controversial subject matter of sexual and reproductive health, serious attention needs to be paid to the approach used to argue the case for support and acceptance. Sometimes, the case may rest primarily on the rights of young people to improved education or services, the reduction of stigma and discrimination, and so on, and research funding may be sought to explore the most effective means of achieving these. Additionally, or alternatively, there may be more pragmatic reasons for action – for example, the threats posed by increasing HIV rates, or the mortality and morbidity associated with illegal abortions – and solutions will be required regarding what can be done about these dilemmas.

A well-developed strategy for presenting a case will have a clear problem statement, defined solutions and will identify and involve key decision makers early on (in the ways described above) to secure political commitment towards getting the results implemented. Among the issues to consider for planning and communication are: Why might the decision-makers be expected to commission and then take on research results? Are there specific issues that have been identified as needing attention? What are the formal and informal needs of the decision-makers? Will the research lead to suggestions for change in policy and/or practice that are realistic, achievable, affordable, likely to address the identified problems?

An important aspect of presenting a strong case for research concerns the methods to be used in the research itself. Some decision-makers are familiar with, and more comfortable with, survey methods using sample populations. While these clearly have their advantages, they are unsuitable for many aspects of the sort of work that is needed when considering young people, marginalised groups and behaviour that may be illegal or sanctioned in other ways. A particularly strong case may need to be made for the use of qualitative methods, both in getting the research funded as well as in getting the results accepted and adopted.

Linking research findings to the government's obligations in law (national law and international human rights treaties) can also be a useful tool for making a case and galvanising wide-ranging support and commitment.

Box 12.2 Trust-building and networking through research leads to new sex education curricula in Nepal

Between 2001 and 2005, the Safe Passages to Adulthood (SPA) team worked with a local NGO, SOLID Nepal, to assist the Government to introduce new sex and relationships education (SRE) curricula in schools in Nepal. This involved a range of strategies.

Research evidence locally owned to underline need for change
International data and new local data were collected that showed poor sexual health among young people, and increasing sexual risk. The research explicitly sought the views of young people and of parents and teachers. The latter groups are traditionally seen as hostile to sex education, but in fact showed strong support for improved SRE curricula in schools. These local data were collected by local researchers who received support and capacity building from SPA. This meant that the results were felt to be locally 'owned'.

Key policy- and decision-makers, as well as young people, involved at all stages
Very early on in the process, a national meeting was organised with key policy personnel as well as young people, parents and teachers to present research findings and discuss opportunities for change. The involvement of young people and parents in the research and dissemination stages was critical to having them on board with the findings and presenting a consensus on the needs and opportunities to the policy representatives. Shortly after this meeting, the Curriculum Development Council (CDC) at the Ministry of Education and Sport requested assistance from SPA's local partner, SOLID Nepal, to develop comprehensive school SRE curricula.

Engaging the media to avoid sensationalism
Concerted efforts were made to involve the national media early on, to brief them fully, to help them understand the issues and concerns, and to try to minimise the risk of sensationalism. Special events, including a three-day workshop, were arranged, and radio and television programmes were planned, as well as newspaper coverage, to try to inform the general public of the need for support. At all times throughout the project, 'traditional values' were openly and sensitively discussed to minimise perceived confrontation. These precautions avoided negative, sensational coverage of the activities and the subsequent curriculum development on a topic that could have been potentially seen as highly threatening to Nepal's traditional cultural values.

External funding, methodological considerations and the importance of context

Engaging with policy- and decision-makers becomes more complex when the research is conceived and funded from outside the country where the research and its findings are expected to be implemented. Most research on young people's sexual and reproductive health in poorer countries is funded from outside the country itself. International agencies, private charitable bodies and bilateral donors support a great deal of the research in the field. This makes the relationships involved somewhat different from those in which the research is commissioned within the country concerned; in this latter case, there may already have been a process of discussion regarding the issues to be addressed, and the funders will be to some extent committed to taking the results seriously, and will almost certainly be closely involved in the process from start to finish.

Where new research has been commissioned from elsewhere, however, or where attempts are to be made to change policy or practice on the basis of research already carried out elsewhere, no such prior relationship can be assumed. In such cases, different strategic approaches will be required. A frequent, but quite misguided, assumption on the part of both researchers and policy-makers is that results obtained in one setting will be easily transferable to a new setting. In reality, research results and their applicability are generally limited to the contexts in which they are obtained, especially for factors as complex as those affecting young people's sexual health.

Of course, the *general issues* and the *questions to be asked* may well be transferable from one site to another; for example, methods used in one area can be used in another (with suitable adaptation where necessary), some of the barriers to change may well exhibit commonalities across countries and be worth exploring in detail (as would be the differences between sites), and the variety of individual reasons for engaging (and/or pressures to engage) in sexual activities can be explored but without assuming that reasons and pressures found in one country will be at all relevant in another. For these, and other reasons, more open-ended research approaches are needed during at least the initial stages of a new research programme.

Practical considerations for researchers

In the light of the complexities of the relationships between decision-makers, researchers, donors and advocates, there are some further practical steps that can be taken to try to maximise the probability of harmonious and fruitful outcomes.

Appropriate levels of research and intervention

In considering the commissioning and application of research in the area of young people's sexual health, some important decisions need to be made regarding the level of intervention that is anticipated. Many studies and associated policy formulations assume that young people themselves are the 'target', and that the task is to understand their shortcomings (such as lack of knowledge, the 'wrong' attitudes to risk, lack of skills to negotiate safety and so on.). While this approach clearly has many merits, there are many other potentially important areas of focus. For example, young people's services will not be successful if the staff display inappropriate attitudes and lack the skills to communicate with their clients. Equally, a new sex and relationships curriculum that might be introduced in schools will fail if the staff charged with delivering it do not feel comfortable with the contents or the style of delivery, or have personal values that conflict with the approach of the programme. These areas are equally worthy of research as is that of the young people themselves.

There will be other levels of research and policy that demand attention over and above the individual levels mentioned above. For example, in places where some of young people's sexual activity can only be fully understood in the context of poverty and the need for income, then effective research and policy change may be directed at income generation schemes rather than directly at sexual activity itself. In areas where there will be strong community opposition to increased attention being given to young people's sexual health, then research to explore the factors that develop and maintain these traditional views may be valuable to enable ways and means to be developed to work with these communities to develop appropriate and acceptable programmes. In these examples, the focus of the work is not so much on young people and risk behaviour in itself, but on the factors that create the contexts in which young people are particularly vulnerable. What is important, whatever the level at which research and policy change are directed, is that there is a clear view of the eventual end product – that is, the improvement of physical and psychological sexual health among young people and the contexts which affect it.

The need for clear guidelines

An essential aspect of the research to policy process, as well as the policy to practice process, is a set of clear and unambiguous guidelines that link the aspects together. A challenge for researchers, and one on which they may need assistance, is translating their findings into realistic and practical implications for policy and programming; for example, a survey finding that many young people do not know of many of the common STIs needs to be accompanied by a set of suggestions as to how this shortfall can be overcome. Having developed a policy to address this shortfall (say, a media campaign, improved sex-and-relationships education in school settings, leaflets and other media for people not in schools, and so on) then practical steps need to be developed to carry out these policies. Intermediary groups, professional communication staff, advertising agencies, and others may all be helpful in making these links and developing suitable guidelines. Again, the value of wide networking with a range of people with specialist skills is stressed.

The importance of dissemination

Researchers located in academic environments tend to use peer refereed journals and book chapters as their main avenues for dissemination; while these are essential for the development of scientific understanding and theo-retical advances, they may be insufficient for effecting policy change. Many in positions of influence within governments and other agencies do not read the academic literature. Intermediaries play a vital function here in 'trans-lating' research findings into language that will be accessible to policy- and decision-makers; equally, however, researchers need to develop skills in communicating to a wide variety of audiences.

One issue that often causes consternation is that research reports are gen-erally quite (or, in some cases, very) long. They may contain appropriate caveats regarding the limits of generalisability, the fine details of some com-plex statistical procedure, some discursive or thematic analysis of qualitative material, and so on. Regrettably, much of this may be simply incomprehensible to some policy-makers who may, as a result, reject the results as being irrelevant and/or too vague to be of practical value. Furthermore, many people in positions of influence are too busy to read long reports, and insist on a short summary, often in the form of an Executive Summary. Much as researchers often dislike seeing the results of their labours (maybe conducted over a two- or three-year period) reduced to a one- or two-page summary, it is often a price that has to be paid if the results are to have an impact.

There are other important avenues for dissemination. Especially in the field of young people and sexual health, the use of the media can be extremely important. Policy is often affected by public opinion, and so the use of selected media can help to inform and persuade the 'general public' of the need for action and help to build pressure for change. Networking with supportive journalists and radio and television staff can pay large dividends, and pieces can be prepared for both the public at large (through national and regional outlets) as well as specific sectors of the population who will have a special interest in the issues – for example, teachers, youth workers, parents, and others – through specialist magazines and programmes.

Increasingly, websites are providing a useful means of disseminating research results and consideration of their implications. For example, the

Alan Guttmacher Institute website contains regular updates and discussions, as does the *Youthnet* programme (see website details below[2]). Access, of course, will be limited in countries and organisations without good computing infrastructures.

It is important not to regard dissemination as something that only happens *after* a research project has been completed. By involving key people throughout the process from start to finish, the chances of successfully ensuring that results are understood and acted upon appropriately can be increased substantially.

Conclusion

The importance of research in informing policy is increasingly recognised. The link between research, policy formulation and practice is complex and demanding, however, and needs to be thought through carefully well in advance. Health and social researchers need a better understanding of the diverse factors that influence policy decisions and processes, and must engage early with a wide range of key players. In this way, they can maximise the opportunities they have for influencing policy in the important and value-laden field of young people's sexual and reproductive health.

Notes

1   Some of the ideas in this chapter derive from a Knowledge Synthesis meeting organised by the *Safe Passages to Adulthood* programme. The meeting involved a mix of researchers, advocates and policy-makers, and focused on their successful and unsuccessful efforts to use research to influence policy in the field of young people's sexual and reproductive health. Those who attended the meeting were Maia Ambegaokar, Peter Aggleton, Andrew Ball, John Ballard, Carlos Cáceres, Mary Crewe, John Cleland, Jacqueline Darroch, Bruce Dick, Ashok Dyalchand, P. Gaye, Roger Ingham, Ana Luisa Liguori, Rachel Partridge, Yasmeen Sabeeh Qazi, George Rae, S. Salinas, Nicole Stone, Waranya Teokul and John Townsend.
2   Alan Guttmacher Institute (www.agi-usguttmacher.org); Youthnet (www.fhi. org/en/youth/youthnet/).

References

Black, N. (2001) Evidence-based policy: Proceed with care, *British Medical Journal*, 323, 275–9.

Brickman, R., Jasanoff, S. and Ilgen, T. (1985) *Controlling Chemicals: The politics of regulation in Europe and the United States*, Ithaca: Cornell University Press.

British Broadcasting Corporation (BBC) (2003) *Vatican in Condom Row*, London: BBC News (available at <www.news.bbc.co.uk/1/hi/health/3176982.stm>).

Buse, K., Mays, N. and Walt, G. (eds) (2005) *Making Health Policy*, Maidenhead: Open University Press.

Cole, J.C., Sumnall, H.R. and Grob, C. (2002) Sorted: Ecstasy, *The Psychologist*, 15(9), 464–7.

Cleland, J. and Ferry B. (eds) (1995) *Sexual Behaviour and AIDS in the Developing World*, London: Taylor and Francis.

Collin, J., Lee, K. and Bissell, K. (2002) The framework convention on tobacco control: The politics of global health governance, *Third World Quarterly*, 23(2), 265–85.

Davis, P. and Howden-Chapman, P. (1996) Translating research findings into health policy, *Social Science and Medicine*, 43(5), 865–72.

Human Rights Watch (2002) *Ignorance Only: HIV/AIDS, human rights and federally funded abstinence-only programs in the United States. Texas – A case study*, HRW, Vol. 14(5) (G) – September 2002.

Human Rights Watch (2005) *The Less They Know The Better: Abstinence-only HIV/AIDS programs in Uganda*, HRW, 17(4) (A) – March 2005.

McKee, M., Garner P. and Stott R. (eds) (2001) *International Co-operation in Health*, Oxford: Oxford University Press.

Miller, D. (1999) Risk, science and policy: Definitional struggles, information management, the media and BSE, *Social Science and Medicine*, 49(9), 1239–55.

Nolan, R. (2002) *Development Anthropology: Encounters in the real world*, Cambridge MA: Westview Press.

Parkhurst, J.O. (2002) The Ugandan success story? Evidence and claims of HIV-1 prevention, *The Lancet*, 360, 78–80.

Peterson M. (2002) Madison Avenue plays a growing role in drug research, *New York Times Online*, <www.nyt.com>.

Rampton, S. and Stauber, J. (2001) *Trust Us, we're Experts: How industry manipulates science and gambles with your future*, New York: Putnam Press.

Russell, A., Sobo, E.J. and Thompson, M.S. (eds) (2000) *Contraception Across Cultures: Technologies, choices, constraints*, Oxford: Berg.

Schneider, H. (2002) On the fault-line: The politics of AIDS policy in contemporary South Africa, *African Studies*, 61(1),145–67.

Trostle, A., Bronfman M. and Langer A. (1999) How do researchers influence decision makers? Case studies from Mexico, *Health Policy and Planning*, 14(2), 103–14.

UN (1989) *UN Convention on the Rights of the Child*, Geneva: UN High Commission for Human Rights.

UN (2003a) *HIV/AIDS and the Rights of the Child*, Committee on the Rights of the Child, thirty-second session (13–31 January 2003), General Comment No. 3, Geneva: United Nations High Commission for Human Rights.

UN (2003b) *Adolescent Health and Development in the Context of the Convention on the Rights of the Child*, Committee on the Rights of the Child, thirty-third session (19 May – 6 June, 2003), General Comment No. 4, Geneva: United Nations High Commission for Human Rights.

US House of Representatives (2004) *The Content of Federally Funded Abstinence-only Education Programs*, Committee on Government Reform – Minority staff special investigations division, report prepared for Rep. Henry A. Waxman, December 2004, Washington DC: US House of Representatives (available at <www.democrats.reform.house.gov/Documents/20041201102153–50247.pdf>).

Walt, G. (1994) *Health Policy: An introduction to process and power*, London: Zed Books.

Index

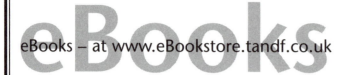